ALSO WRITTEN BY MIRIAM E. NELSON, PH.D.
WITH SARAH WERNICK, PH.D.

Strong Women Stay Young

Strong Women Stay Slim

Strong Women, Strong Bones

WITH JUDY KNIPE

Strong Women Eat Well

AND KRISTIN R. BAKER, PH.D., AND RONENN ROUBENOFF, M.D., M.H.S.
WITH LAWRENCE LINDNER, M.A.

Strong Women and Men Beat Arthritis

The Strong Women's Journal

A 52-WEEK PLANNER TO HELP YOU:

- STAY MOTIVATED

- TRACK PROGRESS

- REACH NUTRITION AND
FITNESS GOALS

Miriam E. Nelson, Ph.D.

Associate Professor, Friedman School of
Nutrition Science and Policy
Tufts University

A PERIGEE BOOK

P

A Perigee Book
Published by The Berkley Publishing Group
A division of Penguin Group (USA) Inc.
375 Hudson Street
New York, New York 10014

Copyright © 2003 by Miriam E. Nelson and Lawrence Lindner
Text design by Richard Oriolo
Cover design by Ben Gibson

First edition: December 2003

THIS BOOK HAS BEEN CATALOGED BY THE LIBRARY OF CONGRESS

Printed in the United States of America
10 9 8 7 6 5 4 3 2

This book is dedicated to
all of the women who have written to me over the years.
Your stories of transformation and triumph have
been an inspiration. Now, in these pages,
they will inspire countless others.

Acknowledgments

USUALLY, A BOOK IS WRITTEN BY ONE, two, or sometimes three people. This one was written by dozens. A very warm thank you to all of the women who graciously gave me permission to use their stories in this journal. I tried very hard to reach each and every one of you. For those stories where I was unable to make contact, I changed the name to protect anonymity. If you are reading this book and find your quote and I was not able to reach you, please contact me, and I will attend to this in future printings.

I'd like to express thanks, too, to my colleagues at Tufts University, *all* of whom have been enormously supportive of my writing efforts. Rebecca Seguin, my project manager at Tufts, provided welcomed assistance in the writing of this book.

To the staff of the *Tufts University Health & Nutrition Letter*, in particular, Larry Lindner, I am grateful for your keen eye, for all the vetting, and for your unflagging logistical support.

My editor, Sheila Curry Oakes, and all of the others at Putnam and Perigee Books, have been dogged promoters of *Strong Women* everywhere. Likewise, I could not have done this work without the support and friendship of my wonderful agent, Wendy Weil.

Neill Walsdorf, Jr., and my colleagues at Mission Pharmacal continue to help me get out the message of good nutrition and exercise for women's health.

Gary Hirshberg, Mary Townsend, and all the others at Stonyfield Farm have been instrumental in promoting *Strong Women*. Much appreciation also goes to the Stonyfield Farm folks for conducting the annual *Strong Women* contest, which has allowed me to benefit from many wonderful stories of women all over the country.

A special note of gratitude to Constance and John Lindner, who gave so generously of their time so that this journal could be completed.

Of course, thank you to all my friends and extended family, who nourish me on the weekends with wonderful food and plenty of fresh air and exercise.

To my immediate family, who nourish me every day—Kin, Mason, Eliza, and Alexandra—thank you for your patience and love.

Contents

The Strong Women's Journal

Introduction: Getting Started

AS WITH MANY OF THE THOUSANDS of strong women who have written to me over the last few years, the following story echoes a common theme: Writing things down helps women take care of themselves as they *become* strong—both emotionally and physically. It keeps them focused and therefore better able to reach their goals.

A decade ago, my dad (my mentor and confidante) died suddenly at 64. I was then diagnosed with a benign tumor, which necessitated the removal of two-thirds of my lung. My brother went through a messy divorce. I had two young daughters and a full-time job. I felt weak and out of control.

I "snapped out of it" by starting with a simple list of things in life that I can control. On the left of a sheet of loose-leaf paper, I listed all the things that made me happy and confident throughout my life (including activities I simply wasn't making time for). On the right were things that consistently made me miserable and stressed—activities, people types, etc.

I started to focus on my left list and indulged in my passions and interests—exercising, healthy eating, reading, writing, my girlfriends, spending time on the beach, time with my daughters, music—awakening in me a strength I had forgotten. I developed the confidence to start a new career and dropped more than 30 pounds. Whenever I'm feeling like the world is overwhelming, I look back at "the list" and am awed by how many positive things I can control in my life and world.

Typically, rather than turn to a single set of lists, women who write things down stay motivated by keeping a journal and tracking their progress as they go along. I'm not at all surprised. I started keeping a journal myself in 1972, when I was 12, and continue to do so today. It's not as detailed as it used to be, but I'm still able to turn to it to help me better understand myself—my feelings and my accomplishments, and whether I've been more or less productive than usual. I can also look back at my exercise and eating patterns to see if I've been getting enough physical activity and choosing the right foods. I can also match my moods to the lapses in the way I take care of myself—and catch myself before I dip too far.

So can Antoinette, someone who wrote to me recently to share her inspirations on how she copes with myriad personal and professional challenges. "Once things are committed to paper," she said, "I am more relaxed—emptying my head and freeing myself to accomplish things instead of worrying about the many things I need to accomplish. This freedom from worry is physically energizing and emotionally exhilarating. Seeing all of my tasks and responsibilities on paper eliminates the anxiety of forgetting both big and small things, allows me to prioritize the importance of everything and everyone demanding my attention, and truly helps me put and keep life in perspective. In short, it allows me to feel more in control of my life; allows me to balance my physical, mental, intellectual, and emotional well-being."

It's not just day-by-day that you measure when you keep a journal; you can also get a sense of how you handle the ebb and flow of the seasons. Because of my diary, I have discovered that I'm simply depressed in February and don't take as good care of myself then as usual. Especially if there's no snow on the ground or the water's not frozen over and I can't enjoy cross-country skiing, skating, or other cold-weather activities, I'm just not myself. Now I don't beat myself up about it; I know that I find the short days and the lack of sunlight in February gloomy, and I've learned to expect less of myself during that time.

I still have all of my journals. They are in a drawer in my bedside table. (I know my kids will have a field day with them when I am gone!) I love going back and reading about my thoughts when I was a teenager and thinking about my first boyfriend; I love going over graphs I used to keep that tracked my monthly cycles and my body temperature while I was in training for races and seeing that I knew I was pregnant with my first child even before I skipped a period because my temperature was elevated; I love going over details of a fantastic hike I took while on a wonderful vacation in France a couple of years ago.

But, as I and many other women know from experience, keeping a journal is much more than a place to moon about boyfriends, explore emotional experiences, or record life events. Research has demonstrated that keeping a journal is a *serious* tool to help keep people committed as they start an exercise and nutrition plan and maintain it over a lifetime. Studies have shown again and again that keeping track of your exercise patterns as well as your dietary choices (both for general health or weight control) is one of the most effective ways of *staying* on track as you make important changes in your lifestyle.

In one study, investigators observed some 2,000 people trying to lose weight. The scientists wanted to see what the successful study volunteers had in common. What they found was that the best predictor for shedding pounds was not, as you might expect, activity level, starting weight, or other such factors but *keeping food records*. The same is true for keeping records when it comes to sticking with an exercise program. In fact, in one of our more recent strength-training studies at Tufts, we encouraged participants to keep written records of how the exercise program was going because we knew it would help people stick with the plan. It did.

Those who maintained a written record got the most out of the program. Even when they didn't accomplish as much as they would have liked, they found it helpful to see their progress—or lack of progress—on paper. It served as a catalogue of what strategies for sticking with the program worked—and which didn't. That, in turn, allowed them to zero in on the things that kept them motivated as well as minimize obstacles that got in their way. Simply being *aware* of obstacles such as time constraints or emotional stress enabled them to strengthen their resolve not to be overcome by roadblocks that might otherwise get them down.

Says one of the many women who have contacted me, "I make sure to write down both short-term and long-term goals, work on them each day, review them regularly, and cross them off as I achieve them. Even if I don't fulfill any particular goal on a given day, knowing that I am a little bit closer gives me the strength to push ahead until I achieve it." As for the motivational aspect, it's exhilarating to look back to where you started and see how far you've come over weeks or months. It shows that even if it sometimes *seems* like things are going too slowly, the momentum worked up over time really does have an impact—more strength gained or more weight lost.

Monitoring your progress in writing also increases your dedication to your goals. If you have to write down every night what you did during the day, you have to answer to yourself for how you spent your time. You have to reckon with whether you let yourself slip for too many days in a row or, perhaps, simply needed a break and let yourself off the hook for a little while because life's stresses were particularly taxing at the time. That happens sometimes, too.

Whatever you discover about yourself, writing it down is a powerful focusing device. It puts your lifestyle activities front and center rather than something you push to the back of your mind. Along with keeping your exercise and eating patterns a priority, it takes pressure off because it turns long-term goals that are difficult to get your arms around into short-term goals that you can hold in your hand. A woman named Louisa who puts her long-range goals on paper likens it to cutting a plan "into bite-size pieces and taking it one bite at a time." That is, if you write it down day by day, you are making frequent notes to yourself about whether you've strength trained, or eaten five fruits and vegetables, or done some aerobic exercise. If you miss your goals for a day or two, or even for a whole month, you can see that it's not a complete slide but just a short-lived lapse. And owning up to the lapse, especially in writing, offers you an opportunity to rededicate yourself to your goals. When you don't write it down, on the other hand, one day turns into the next, and so on, until all your good intentions *can* very easily slip further and further away from you.

That's where the *Strong Women's Journal* comes in. Not only will each day in this 52-week record keeper leave room for you to make long-term plans and jot down your thoughts and feelings—"drain your brain," as a woman wrote to me. Each day will also be set up so that you can quickly, in just a minute or two, keep daily track of whether you're meeting minimum daily exercise and nutrition goals: specifically, taking part in at least 30 minutes of physical activity on most days of the week; strength training two or three times a week; and eating the right amounts of produce, dairy products, whole grains, and so on.

How to Use This Journal

As you read the following sections, take a look at the sample days I filled out for the week of March 22. It'll give you a clear idea of exactly how the journal is set up—and why the format, which I designed with efficiency in mind, requires only a few minutes of your time each day.

Personal Notes

Each week of the *Strong Women's Journal*, which can stand alone or serve as a companion guide for any of my other five books in the *Strong Women* series, starts with a Personal Notes section for putting your thoughts and emotions (and perhaps your short-term goals) on paper every day. This section also has a box each day for rating your mood, vigor, and sleep quality so that you can discern patterns over time. You may see that when your mood and energy level are higher, for instance, you're more inclined to take better care of yourself.

Along with checking off your sleep quality and the information in other boxes each day, do try to make full use of Personal Notes by taking a couple of minutes to write a few lines. Comments a *Strong Women* reader named Leigh Anne, "Regular journal entries are how I stay strong every day. Although my days are packed with career and personal concerns, I scribble my thoughts down. If I'm worried or annoyed about something, writing it down helps me get it out of my system and get on with my day. Sometimes I list the aspects of my life for which I'm grateful. Occasionally, I vent about problems that might seem petty if I mentioned them out loud. Putting my emotions onto the page helps me feel better and gain perspective. The biggest plus—nobody ever has to read it except me, so I don't have to worry about holding back! You don't have to be Jane Austen or Virginia Woolf. You don't have to write neatly or in complete sentences, and spelling is definitely NOT a factor. What matters most is that you express yourself in words that reflect how you feel and think at the moment. Who knows? Once you start, you may find yourself brainstorming brilliant ideas for your next major life project. A personal journal has helped me get to the heart of who I am."

Sleep—As Important as Exercise and Eating Right

◈

Sleep is crucial to success, which is why I feel it's so important that you track it. A friend and correspondent, Jenny, drove home the importance of restful slumber when she wrote to me, "Fatigue is the enemy. Fatigue and its handmaiden, stress, rob the body of stamina and the mind of spirit." That's why, even though Jenny has her share of daily demands with two children and a full work life, she makes sure to get a good night's sleep on top of exercising every day and eating well. "It's not selfish," she says, "but a winning strategy for boosting energy so that you can face any challenge and offer the world all that you can." I'm with Jenny all the way on this. My whole family puts a high value on sleep—even my teenagers! We're all in bed before 10 o'clock on most nights.

To improve the quality and quantity of your own sleep:

- Avoid caffeine, nicotine, and alcohol at least 4 hours before bedtime. Caffeine and nicotine are stimulants that in the body take a relatively long time to break down. And alcohol, while it helps initiate sleep, interferes with deep sleep later on in the night and can cause awakenings.

- Don't stay in bed for more than 15 or 20 minutes of not being able to sleep. Go to another room to read or watch television, and return to bed only when you feel tired enough to sleep.

- Don't engage in something before bed that will give you a second wind, like watching an action-packed movie.

- Keep your bedroom at a comfortable temperature. A room that's too hot or too cold can keep you awake.

- Use your bedroom only for sleep and sex rather than treating it like a second family room with a TV and computer.

- Stick to a schedule, waking up pretty much the same time on weekends as during the week.

If you're having trouble falling asleep, try soaking in a hot bath or taking a hot shower. It can help bring on sleep by relaxing tense muscles.

Another freedom you can take writing in your journal besides venting your feelings without worrying about spelling or grammar is that you don't have to use January 1 as a start date. Sometimes a move toward a new goal is marked by a date entirely unrelated to New Year's. For instance, someone not long ago communicated to me that "July 6 is an important anniversary for me. Six years ago, I began the exercise program that has become an important part of my life. At the time, I had two children from a previous marriage, had remarried, and had a lovely baby boy. However, I was feeling the stress of the new marriage, children finishing high school, and a newborn. My son's day-care provider and I decided to make an exercise date every day. We started walking each day after work. . . ."

Any day of the year can mark the beginning of change for you. If you don't pick this journal up in January but do so in May, turn to the exact date that you bring it home and start there. Work forward through December 31, then flip back to January 1 when it's time and keep going until you have all 12 months filled in and you're back to your start date. No matter where you begin, you'll still be able to see all of your steps build to great success, and you'll discover the patterns in your way of life that continually lead you to new solutions. You don't need to wait for New Year's to take on a new goal. Whatever date you start is the right one.

Nutrition Log

The weekly Personal Notes pages are followed by a weekly Nutrition Log, which will let you see at a glance whether you are keeping up day-to-day with specific goals for how much of which foods to eat. (See Daily Nutrition Goals box.) The Nutrition Log also leaves room to jot down some notes about your eating pattern each day. Use the space for notes however it suits you. One person may want to keep track of every single food she eats. Another may only want to track how she controls her food choices and portion sizes when she eats out. While I do a combination of the two, some days I don't write any notes. If I'm super busy, I just check off the boxes for my daily goals. Use the Notes section however it's going to help you most to track and achieve your nutrition goals.

The goals in the Daily Nutrition Goals box, based on the latest research on nutrition and health promotion, may look to you like an updated version of the government's Food Guide Pyramid (which is currently under reconstruction itself). But there are a few significant differences, which I feel are crucial for the best nutrition guidance possible. A number of them have to do with "Extras," which is another term for "Use sparingly."

You will see an "Extras" box in the Nutrition Log. What I consider extras departs

Daily Nutrition Goals

൦ൔඁ

- At least three servings of whole-grain foods (one serving = a 1-ounce slice of bread; 1 ounce of breakfast cereal; ½ cup cooked cereal, rice, pasta, or other grain; or ¾ cup cold cereal. In this section, record only whole grains.

- At least two servings of fruit (one serving = 1 medium apple, banana, or orange; ½ cup chopped (raw, cooked, or canned) fruit; ¾ cup fruit juice (not fruit juice *beverage* or *drink*, which won't be 100% fruit juice).

- At least three servings of vegetables (one serving = 1 cup raw leafy greens; ½ cup other vegetables, cooked; ¾ cup vegetable juice).

- Two to four servings of protein-rich foods (one serving = 3 ounces cooked fish, beef, poultry, or pork; ½ cup cooked dry beans; ½ cup soybeans or tofu; 1 egg; 2 tablespoons peanut butter; or ½–1 ounce nuts).

- Two to three dairy servings (one serving = 1 cup milk or yogurt, preferably low- or nonfat) 1½ ounces hard cheese, such as Swiss or Cheddar—soft cheeses have less calcium.

significantly from what are traditionally considered extras. For instance, potatoes come under extras rather than vegetables because even though they contain nutrients like vitamin C and potassium and their skins have fiber, they consist of too much starch—and therefore too many calories—to be thought of as a vegetable in the same way as produce like spinach and broccoli. You should also record in the extras box each sugary, fatty food or beverage that doesn't have a lot of nutrients for its calories. That includes cakes, cookies, ice cream, candy bars, potato chips, French fries, sugary soda pop, and alcoholic drinks.

Record high-fat items such as butter and sour cream as extras, too. But, contrary to popular belief, not every single fat is an extra. Numerous findings have shown that the highly unsaturated fats in fish and certain nuts, for example, called omega-3 fatty acids, are an essential part of the diet. They are widely thought to help ward off and control the course of such illnesses as heart disease and arthritis. Because of the benefits of omega-

3 fatty acids, the American Heart Association says that everyone should strive to eat at least two fish meals a week. Flaxseed oil also has omega-3s, as does canola oil.

Omega-3s from nuts and other non-fish sources aren't used as efficiently by the body to minimize the risk of disease, but they are much, much better for your health than the saturated fats found in butter, whole-milk dairy products, and fatty cuts of meat. Saturated fats raise blood cholesterol and thereby increase the risk for heart disease. So do trans fats, which are found in everything from snack foods to desserts. (Trans fats are listed in the ingredients as "hydrogenated oil" or "partially hydrogenated oil.")

Of course, even though healthful omega-3s are not extras, that doesn't mean you should go overboard on them. All fat, no matter what the source, has about 120 calories a tablespoon. (An ounce of nuts has between 150 and 200 calories.) But you should judiciously incorporate sources of omega-3s into your diet while cutting back on sources of saturated and trans fats.

Just as not all fats are extras, not all grains belong in the Grains group. Any grains that are not whole-grain, including white bread, bagels, white rice, regular pasta, and non-whole-grain breakfast cereals, should be considered extras.

I'm not anti-carbohydrate or a proponent of the very high-protein, high-fat diets that tell you to eschew carbohydrates altogether. After all, fruits and vegetables are largely carbohydrate, and studies across the board show that they promote health. I also enjoy a bowl of pasta now and then, just like the next person. But many people eat much more in the way of *refined* carbohydrates than is consistent with a healthful dietary pattern and weight management goals. More to the point, whole-grain foods are so much more healthful than refined. They are higher in fiber and a host of nutrients, including zinc, magnesium, manganese, potassium, copper, vitamin E, vitamin B$_6$, and the B vitamin pantothenic acid. They are also higher in phytochemicals that researchers are only now discovering may play a crucial role in warding off disease. Whole-grain phytochemicals called lignans, for example, may protect against cancers that are hormonally influenced, including breast cancer.

Studies have shown, too, a strong correlation between eating diets high in whole grains and enjoying a reduced risk for some of the major illnesses that plague women and men today. Harvard's Nurses' Health Study, which follows tens of thousands of women, has indicated a link between consumption of whole grains and a reduced risk for developing type 2 diabetes. The Iowa Women's Health Study, which keeps tabs on the diets of more than 30,000 women, makes the same association. Research on both groups of women also suggests that whole grains protect against heart disease.

Unfortunately, only about five percent of the grain-based foods in the typical American supermarket are whole grain, so you've got to look hard. Check breads and breakfast cereals to make sure the first term on the ingredients list is "whole grain" or "whole wheat" or "oats" or "whole rolled oats." Terms like "unbromated flour," "unbleached flour," "7-grain," and "multi-grain" don't cut it. Unless the product is made from oats, the word "whole" has to come first.

To vary your whole-grain repertoire, consider trying one with your dinner instead of rice or pasta, which are usually eaten in their refined, white versions. Following is a chart of different types of whole-grain foods, with approximate cooking times, that you can generally find either in your supermarket rice aisle or natural foods section. (Another good bet is one of the newer, larger natural foods supermarkets.) The yield for each after cooking is about four cups. Remember, one cup is two servings from the grains group.

WHOLE GRAIN	AMT. OF LIQUID NEEDED FOR 1 CUP OF GRAIN	COOKING TIME
Barley (quick, not pearled)	1¾ cups	15–18 mins
Buckwheat groats (also called kasha)	2 cups	5–7 mins
Bulgur	1½–2 cups	15–20 mins
Millet	2¼–2¾ cups	25–30 mins
Quinoa (pronounced KEEN-wah)	2 cups	15–20 mins
Wheatberries, spelt, or faro (soaked overnight)	2½–3 cups	30 mins

A final point here on extras: Having a few cookies here or there or even a small piece of chocolate or butter every single day is not going to wreck your diet. In fact, it can add a great deal of pleasure. But if your diet is heavy on extras at the expense of more nutritious foods, you'll want to rethink—and adjust—your overall eating pattern.

Note that the bottom of the Nutrition Log leaves room to check off whether you've taken a daily calcium tablet or other supplement or incorporated a particular food into your meals for its health properties. All women capable of becoming pregnant should consider taking a multivitamin with folate to reduce the chance of having a baby with a neural tube defect. And I recommend that women over the age of 35 take 500 to 700 mg of supplemental calcium (preferably calcium citrate) daily as well as 400 to 600 IU of vitamin D to protect their bones. In addition, some women take vitamin E because evidence suggests it helps immune function. Then there are the more individual decisions about supplements. For instance, I add 2 teaspoons of omega-3–rich flaxseed oil to my yogurt several days a week (about 80 calories' worth). As I outline above, this is not an extra but an item I choose to include in my diet for potential disease prevention.

Finally, the Nutrition Log leaves room for Overall Comments so that after discerning a pattern, you can note to yourself, say, that you need to be eating more vegetables or fewer extras.

Exercise Log

After each weekly Nutrition Log comes a weekly exercise page, which is separated into Physical Activity (which targets your heart and lungs as well as flexibility and coordination) and Strength Training (which maintains and strengthens your muscle mass and bone—so crucial for keeping back the frailty that otherwise begins to accrue from the time a woman is in her mid-forties).

Physical activity can be any combination of planned aerobic activities like brisk walking, jogging, or swimming laps; sports such as tennis; dancing or heavy-duty gardening; errands (such as walking to the store for milk instead of driving); games like badminton in the backyard; or flexibility and coordination exercises such as tai chi and yoga. The goal here is to get 30 to 60 minutes of such activity on most, if not all, days of the week, so there's a slot for you to write in your time each day.

Strength training, for maximum gain without risk of injury, should be performed two to three times a week—with at least one day between sessions. You should perform six to 12 exercises during a session, some focusing on the upper body (such as the biceps curl or side arm raise); some focusing on the lower body (such as the knee extension or step-up); and some focusing on the trunk (such as abdominal curls or back extensions). In the Exercise Log, record the amount of weight you lifted or, if that's not applicable, a check mark (✓).

The American College of Sports Medicine encourages people to do one to three "sets" of each exercise, with six to 15 repetitions per set. I think this is a reasonable recommendation, but my own experience is that for maximum efficiency and effectiveness, two sets, each with eight to 10 repetitions, is good. There should also be about a minute of rest between sets. (For more information on the specifics on how to perform strength-training exercises, consult *Strong Women Stay Young*, *Strong Women Stay Slim*, *Strong Women, Strong Bones*, or *Strong Women and Men Beat Arthritis*. Each, as their titles suggest, emphasizes a different aspect of strength training.)

Note: Some women like to break up their strength training into six shorter sessions on six different days: two days for the upper body, two for the lower, and two for the trunk. That's fine, as long as you don't exercise any one part of the body two days in a row.

You will see that the bottom of the exercise page has a place for you to write down how many steps you take each day. Far and away the most common activity that people do on a daily basis is walking. I highly recommend that you wear a pedometer to keep track. Health experts say that optimally, you should be getting 10,000 steps each day, and I agree. You might not always reach 10,000; it comes to about 4.5 miles accumulated over the course of the day. But whether or not you get to that level on a regular basis, a pedometer is a great motivator. Once you have a number, you have a goal—to increase it.

Make sure that you follow the manufacturer's directions when wearing the device. Also, keep in mind that you don't need a fancy one. I like the ones that just count steps and nothing more. They cost $20 to $30. See "Resources" at the back of the book for where to buy pedometers.

Below are sample pages that I kept for a week in March.

MARCH 22–28

PERSONAL NOTES

MARCH 22, DAY OF THE WEEK S M T W TH F (S)

Had a lazy morning with a delicious waffle breakfast. Took a walk with Regina. Spring is starting to show some signs. In the afternoon we all went to the rock gym. Mason is so much fun to watch. Stopped at the mall to pick up a few clothes for the kids. Watched "To Kill a Mockingbird" tonight with the kids—What a powerful movie.

	MOOD	VIGOR	SLEEP
Excellent	✓	✓	✓
	☐	☐	☐
	☐	☐	☐
Poor			

MARCH 23, DAY OF THE WEEK (S) M T W TH F S

Worked in the yard with Kin for a couple of hours this morning trying to start the long clean-up after this severe Winter. Alexandra had soccer practice. Finished our taxes—Ugh! Strength trained at home. Took a quick run with Eliza. Helped the kids with homework and went to bed early.

	MOOD	VIGOR	SLEEP
Excellent	✓	✓	✓
	☐	☐	☐
	☐	☐	☐
Poor			

MARCH 24, DAY OF THE WEEK S (M) T W TH F S

Took the train. Had a good day at work. Talked with folks in Alaska and Kansas about the upcoming Strong Women Conference. I am eager to get them trained so that they can start some community programs. They seem very excited. Otherwise just wrote and worked on the grant.

	MOOD	VIGOR	SLEEP
Excellent	☐	✓	✓
	✓	☐	☐
	☐	☐	☐
Poor			

MARCH 25, DAY OF THE WEEK S M (T) W TH F S

Seemed to have conference call and interview one after another today. I didn't get as much done as I would have liked. Need to manage my time better. I need to carve out a least 3 hours a day where I don't take calls or get an email. Alexandra had a soccer game tonight—scored the winning goal with one minute left—very exciting!

	MOOD	VIGOR	SLEEP
Excellent	☐	☐	✓
	✓	✓	☐
	☐	☐	☐
Poor			

MARCH 22–28

PERSONAL NOTES

MARCH 26, DAY OF THE WEEK S M T (W) TH F S

Took the train. Dr. Rosenberg and Sue Lautze gave the seminar today
on the development of a national nutrition program in Afghanistan—
fascinating! Had my first crown put in today. It seemed like the drilling
would never stop. I am pretty sore. Worked on the grant. Did a yoga tape
when I got home. It helped me relax and not concentrate on my tooth.

MOOD	VIGOR	SLEEP
Excellent		
☐	☐	✓
✓	☐	☐
☐	✓	☐
Poor		

MARCH 27, DAY OF THE WEEK S M T W (TH) F S

Had several meetings today but was able to carve out a chunk of
uninterrupted time this morning for solid writing. Had a meeting with my
Omidyar Scholars this afternoon in Medford. They are really doing well. We
are getting some great ideas on how to improve the food served at Restaurants
in Somerville for the Shape Up Somerville project. Strength trained.

MOOD	VIGOR	SLEEP
Excellent		
✓	✓	☐
☐	☐	✓
☐	☐	☐
Poor		

MARCH 28, DAY OF THE WEEK S M T W TH (F) S

Worked at home today. Prepared my talk for Rhode Island tomorrow. Had
a couple of interviews. Ran at lunch. Went to the rock gym this evening
with all the kids and a few extras—feel strong. Eliza is really getting
strong. I love to watch her climb. I love my kids. Kin and I really need to
work on having a little more time to ourselves—Agreed next week we will
go out to dinner together.

MOOD	VIGOR	SLEEP
Excellent		
✓	✓	✓
☐	☐	☐
☐	☐	☐
Poor		

MARCH 22–28
NUTRITION LOG

GOALS (# SERVINGS)	WHOLE GRAINS 3+	FRUITS 2+	VEGETABLES 3+	PROTEIN 2–4	DAIRY 2–3	EXTRAS VARIABLE
MARCH 22	4	2	3	4	2	3

NOTES: *Waffles with fruit, OJ, yogurt and almonds, tuna salad sandwich on whole wheat, banana, cheese and crackers, carrot, tofu, veggies, brown rice, ice cream, 1/2 beer*

MARCH 23	3	3	4	4	3	3

NOTES:

MARCH 24	3	3	3	4	3	4

NOTES: *Went to O'Naturals after Alexandra's soccer game*

MARCH 25	4	3	3	4	3	4

NOTES:

MARCH 26	2	2	4	3	2	2

NOTES: *Mouth hurt today because of Crown*

MARCH 27	4	2	3	4	2	3

NOTES:

MARCH 28	3	3	3	4	3	4

NOTES: *Had a nice lunch at home with Kin*

CALCIUM + VITAMIN D ✔ VITAMIN E ✔ MULTIVITAMIN/MINERAL ☐

PLENTY OF FLUIDS ☐ OTHER SUPPLEMENTS *flaxseed oil*

OVERALL COMMENTS *Work on drinking more fluids; need to eat slower at lunch*

PHYSICAL ACTIVITY

planned, sport, leisure, errands, play
Goal: 30 to 60 minutes most days of the week

DAY	ACTIVITY	TIME
3/22	Walk with Regina	1 hour
3/22	Rock gym	1:30
3/23	Yard work	2 hours
3/24	Took train + walked to work	total 45 min
3/26	Took train + walked to work	total 45 min
3/26	Yoga tape	30 min
3/27	Walked from Subway to Campus	45 min
3/28	Run	35 min
3/28	Rock gym	1:30

STRENGTH TRAINING

Goal: 2 to 3 times per week

EXERCISE 2 SETS/8 TO 10 REPS	DAY: 3/23 POUNDS OR ✓	DAY: 3/25 POUNDS OR ✓	DAY: 3/27 POUNDS OR ✓
Biceps curl	12		12
Overhead press	10		10
Side arm raise	6		6
Knee extension	15		15
Knee curl	10		~~10~~ 9
Squats		✓	
Step-ups		✓	
Ab crunches		✓	
Back extensions		✓	
Pull-ups	✓		✓

NUMBER OF STEPS

MARCH 22	MARCH 23	MARCH 24	MARCH 25	MARCH 26	MARCH 27	MARCH 28
13,481	12,530	10,823	7,822	10,181	11,280	9,784

MONTHLY REVIEW

At the end of each month is space for a monthly review so that you can begin to track your progress over longer stretches of time. You'll want to fill in your bright spots for that month as well as your greatest challenges, looking for patterns to see what gets you to your goals and what keeps you from them. This will allow you to identify barriers to change, both personal and professional, and steer you toward clues for how to overcome them.

I also think it's important for you to take a few minutes at the end of each month to see that you're paying attention to personal care: flossing, keeping your skin moisturized, and, for some women, having your hair styled, cut, or colored when necessary. (Keeping well groomed is part of taking care of yourself.) In addition, I'll ask you to check whether you've had any sick days or simply have not been feeling your best. You'll want to record your weight, too, days of your menstrual cycle (if applicable), whether you've seen the doctor or dentist, and any medications you've taken. Focusing on these aspects of your life is a good way of determining whether you're attending to basic maintenance, in the same way you get an oil and filter change every so often in order to get the most out of your car.

Once-a-month weighing definitely works for me. I used to weigh myself only about once a year. But a couple of years ago, my thyroid started giving me problems. I lost about 15 pounds (without wanting to) before it was stabilized, and I was able to gain back the weight. Now, to make sure things don't slip, I get on the scale once a month. Weighing yourself every day is not recommended because you'll just see water shifts. Even once a week is not necessary, but some women find it helpful in programs such as Weight Watchers. Certainly, once a month lets you keep track of your health over time.

KEEPING YOURSELF WELL: MEDICAL SCREENINGS

From day to day, you're the one in charge of keeping yourself healthy and productive. But there are some things you need your doctor to help you keep track of: whether your cholesterol and blood pressure are in the normal range, for example; whether your bone density requires you to take extra precautions against fractures; whether your thyroid gland requires medication to keep working properly (a relatively frequent need for women over 35); and so on. That's why, on pages 274–275, I list the basic medical screening tests you'll need at some point(s) in your life. The list is a jumping-off point for discussions with your doctor about when you'll need which tests, and it will allow you to easily check off whether you're following through appropriately on routine health care.

THE YEAR IN REVIEW

The last part of this journal, to be filled in after you have gone through an entire year, contains a series of questions to ask yourself as you look over 12 months' worth of entries. Some of them are very basic: Did you meet the basic nutrition goals? Did you increase the amount of weight that you lifted over the year? Did you stretch after workouts? But some are more probing: In which month(s) did you achieve your greatest accomplishments? Which month(s) were the most difficult? Taking some time to carefully consider the answers to these questions will allow you to look at the bigger cyclical picture over time, not just day-to-day. It will also help you devise strategies to get around obstacles. For instance, a woman can take a motivating principle from a month that worked out really well in order to improve months that she knows historically are difficult.

May is always a good month for me, and I use it as inspiration for how to eat well in February, when I tend to feel down and therefore need more self-prodding to eat right. I tell myself in mid-winter that while I can't get the summer vegetables I enjoy most, it is important to eat healthfully and make an effort to buy what *is* in season—delicious, nutrient-rich winter squash, for instance, and all kinds of apples—from tart to sweet to crunchy to soft. I also look for good-quality frozen produce, and I can eat more dried fruit. In addition, I buy some things out of season that I enjoy, even though it might be more expensive and goes against my desire to buy locally produced products.

But I'm just one person with one set of experiences and ideas. Difficult people have various solutions and suggestions of their own that you may find useful. That's why, throughout the journal, you will find tips and inspirations from dozens and dozens of the many women who have contacted me over the years. As you fill in your own pages, you'll find advice from these women on everything from how to talk yourself through a rough patch to how to add fruits and vegetables to your meals—easily. One nutrition-savvy woman pointed out that if you make a sandwich with spinach leaves instead of lettuce leaves, you'll get 11 percent more of the Daily Value for folate and 40 percent more for vitamin A!

In a dozen larger essays—one for each month—you'll learn strategies for overcoming obstacles ("I don't have time") to breaking goals into small steps ("The Power of Progression") to nourishing intimacy (which can come unexpectedly and in many forms, from coworkers and friends as well as spouses). There's even information on how some women use the strategy of visualization to shepherd themselves toward their goals, while others participate in volunteer work because being an agent of change for others grounds them and strengthens them in their own efforts as they go forward.

I hope this book serves as an agent of change for *you*—whether it helps you eat better; exercise more consistently; learn how to say "no" (see November); de-stress (August); see that moving forward sometimes involves what seems like moving backward (April); or take a leap of faith that living strong one day at a time will get you to your goals, even if a change feels uncomfortable or like a "drop in the bucket" at first.

Wishing you a strong today and an even better tomorrow,

Miriam

GOAL SETTING

You are about to change your life. Before you start, you need to think about what you want to accomplish over the next year, not just health-wise but also in your personal and professional life. Consider your major goals, and then think hard about how you are going to accomplish them. That is, what are the concrete and specific short-term goals that are going to help you reach your long-term ones? For instance, if your overall aim is to lose weight, will you limit sweets to once a day? Walk at least four miles every other day? This small investment in time to come up with targeted behavior changes rather than just lists of how you ultimately want to look or feel will help you throughout the year. Also, remember that your goals can change—so don't hesitate to update this page if necessary.

MAJOR GOALS:

Nutrition   *Eat healthier*

How am I going to accomplish them?

Eat more fruits + veggies

Physical activity   *Be stronger, more fit.*

How am I going to accomplish them?

Do strength training 2-3x per week along w/ walking.

Personal   *Have a strong network of friends.*

How am I going to accomplish them?

Reach out more.

Professional

How am I going to accomplish them?

Start my Life Coaching Business.

If weight loss is your goal, try this simple rule: Don't eat after 8 p.m. In a study in Sweden, researchers found that obese woman ate the same amount of food as healthy-weight women for most of the day but piled on extra calories from 8 p.m. until midnight. (They also tended to eat more from 2 to 4 p.m.)

JANUARY 18, DAY OF THE WEEK   S   M   T   W   TH   F   S

MOOD	VIGOR	SLEEP
Excellent		
☐	☐	☐
☐	☐	☐
☐	☐	☐
Poor		

JANUARY 19, DAY OF THE WEEK   S   M   T   W   TH   F   S

MOOD	VIGOR	SLEEP
Excellent		
☐	☐	☐
☐	☐	☐
☐	☐	☐
Poor		

JANUARY 20, DAY OF THE WEEK   S   M   T   W   TH   F   S

MOOD	VIGOR	SLEEP
Excellent		
☐	☐	☐
☐	☐	☐
☐	☐	☐
Poor		

JANUARY 21, DAY OF THE WEEK   S   M   T   W   TH   F   S

MOOD	VIGOR	SLEEP
Excellent		
☐	☐	☐
☐	☐	☐
☐	☐	☐
Poor		

JANUARY 15–21
NUTRITION LOG

GOALS (# SERVINGS)	WHOLE GRAINS 3+	FRUITS 2+	VEGETABLES 3+	PROTEIN 2–4	DAIRY 2–3	EXTRAS VARIABLE
JANUARY 15	☐	☐	☐	☐	☐	☐
NOTES:						
JANUARY 16	☐	☐	☐	☐	☐	☐
NOTES:						
JANUARY 17	☐	☐	☐	☐	☐	☐
NOTES:						
JANUARY 18	☐	☐	☐	☐	☐	☐
NOTES:						
JANUARY 19	☐	☐	☐	☐	☐	☐
NOTES:						
JANUARY 20	☐	☐	☐	☐	☐	☐
NOTES:						
JANUARY 21	☐	☐	☐	☐	☐	☐
NOTES:						

CALCIUM + VITAMIN D ☐ **VITAMIN E** ☐ **MULTIVITAMIN/MINERAL** ☐

PLENTY OF FLUIDS ☐ **OTHER SUPPLEMENTS** _____

OVERALL COMMENTS

PHYSICAL ACTIVITY

planned, sport, leisure, errands, play
Goal: 30 to 60 minutes most days of the week

DAY	ACTIVITY	TIME

STRENGTH TRAINING

Goal: 2 to 3 times per week

EXERCISE 2 SETS/8 TO 10 REPS	DAY: POUNDS OR ✓	DAY: POUNDS OR ✓	DAY: POUNDS OR ✓

NUMBER OF STEPS

JANUARY 15	JANUARY 16	JANUARY 17	JANUARY 18	JANUARY 19	JANUARY 20	JANUARY 21

January 22–28

Recently, I hiked the Long Trail through Vermont, from the Massachusetts border to Canada. In four weeks I walked more than 260 miles of rugged terrain. The key to my success was taking a maxi-goal and approaching it on a mini-level. On a daily basis, it was simple: walk from point A to point B. With patience and drive, no task is insurmountable.—Anonymous

Personal Notes

JANUARY 22, DAY OF THE WEEK S M T W TH F S

MOOD	VIGOR	SLEEP
Excellent		
☐	☐	☐
☐	☐	☐
☐	☐	☐
Poor		

JANUARY 23, DAY OF THE WEEK S M T W TH F S

MOOD	VIGOR	SLEEP
Excellent		
☐	☐	☐
☐	☐	☐
☐	☐	☐
Poor		

JANUARY 24, DAY OF THE WEEK S M T W TH F S

MOOD	VIGOR	SLEEP
Excellent		
☐	☐	☐
☐	☐	☐
☐	☐	☐
Poor		

Plan a vacation. Psychologists who followed more than 12,000 people at risk for heart disease found that those who took more vacations during a 5-year study had a 17 percent lower risk of dying during the following decade than those who got away less often. A little R&R is crucial to your health.

JANUARY 25, DAY OF THE WEEK   S   M   T   W   TH   F   S

MOOD	VIGOR	SLEEP
	Excellent	
☐	☐	☐
☐	☐	☐
☐	☐	☐
	Poor	

JANUARY 26, DAY OF THE WEEK   S   M   T   W   TH   F   S

MOOD	VIGOR	SLEEP
	Excellent	
☐	☐	☐
☐	☐	☐
☐	☐	☐
	Poor	

JANUARY 27, DAY OF THE WEEK   S   M   T   W   TH   F   S

MOOD	VIGOR	SLEEP
	Excellent	
☐	☐	☐
☐	☐	☐
☐	☐	☐
	Poor	

JANUARY 28, DAY OF THE WEEK   S   M   T   W   TH   F   S

MOOD	VIGOR	SLEEP
	Excellent	
☐	☐	☐
☐	☐	☐
☐	☐	☐
	Poor	

JANUARY 22–28
NUTRITION LOG

GOALS (# SERVINGS)	WHOLE GRAINS 3+	FRUITS 2+	VEGETABLES 3+	PROTEIN 2–4	DAIRY 2–3	EXTRAS VARIABLE
JANUARY 22 NOTES:	☐	☐	☐	☐	☐	☐
JANUARY 23 NOTES:	☐	☐	☐	☐	☐	☐
JANUARY 24 NOTES:	☐	☐	☐	☐	☐	☐
JANUARY 25 NOTES:	☐	☐	☐	☐	☐	☐
JANUARY 26 NOTES:	☐	☐	☐	☐	☐	☐
JANUARY 27 NOTES:	☐	☐	☐	☐	☐	☐
JANUARY 28 NOTES:	☐	☐	☐	☐	☐	☐

CALCIUM + VITAMIN D ☐   VITAMIN E ☐   MULTIVITAMIN/MINERAL ☐

PLENTY OF FLUIDS ☐   OTHER SUPPLEMENTS _____

OVERALL COMMENTS

PHYSICAL ACTIVITY

planned, sport, leisure, errands, play
Goal: 30 to 60 minutes most days of the week

DAY	ACTIVITY	TIME

STRENGTH TRAINING

Goal: 2 to 3 times per week

EXERCISE 2 SETS/8 TO 10 REPS	DAY: POUNDS OR ✓	DAY: POUNDS OR ✓	DAY: POUNDS OR ✓

NUMBER OF STEPS

JANUARY 22	JANUARY 23	JANUARY 24	JANUARY 25	JANUARY 26	JANUARY 27	JANUARY 28

January 29–31

Personal Notes

JANUARY 29, DAY OF THE WEEK   S   M   T   W   TH   F   S

MOOD	VIGOR	SLEEP
Excellent		
☐	☐	☐
☐	☐	☐
☐	☐	☐
Poor		

JANUARY 30, DAY OF THE WEEK   S   M   T   W   TH   F   S

MOOD	VIGOR	SLEEP
Excellent		
☐	☐	☐
☐	☐	☐
☐	☐	☐
Poor		

JANUARY 31, DAY OF THE WEEK   S   M   T   W   TH   F   S

MOOD	VIGOR	SLEEP
Excellent		
☐	☐	☐
☐	☐	☐
☐	☐	☐
Poor		

JANUARY 29–31
NUTRITION LOG

GOALS (# SERVINGS)	WHOLE GRAINS	FRUITS	VEGETABLES	PROTEIN	DAIRY	EXTRAS
	3+	2+	3+	2–4	2–3	VARIABLE
JANUARY 29	☐	☐	☐	☐	☐	☐
NOTES:						
JANUARY 30	☐	☐	☐	☐	☐	☐
NOTES:						
JANUARY 31	☐	☐	☐	☐	☐	☐
NOTES:						

CALCIUM + VITAMIN D ☐   VITAMIN E ☐   MULTIVITAMIN/MINERAL ☐

PLENTY OF FLUIDS ☐   OTHER SUPPLEMENTS _____

OVERALL COMMENTS

PHYSICAL ACTIVITY

planned, sport, leisure, errands, play
Goal: 30 to 60 minutes most days of the week

DAY	ACTIVITY	TIME

STRENGTH TRAINING

Goal: 2 to 3 times per week

EXERCISE 2 SETS/8 TO 10 REPS	DAY: POUNDS OR ✓	DAY: POUNDS OR ✓	DAY: POUNDS OR ✓

NUMBER OF STEPS

JANUARY 29   JANUARY 30   JANUARY 31

_____   _____   _____

JANUARY REVIEW

BRIGHT SPOTS:

_____

GREATEST CHALLENGES:

_____

_____

PATTERNS OBSERVED:

_____

IDENTIFY BARRIERS TO CHANGE AND HOW I AM GOING TO OVERCOME THEM:

PERSONAL

_____

_____

PROFESSIONAL

_____

_____

PERSONAL CARE ATTENTION (flossing teeth, skin care, cutting/coloring hair, etc.):

_____

_____

WELLNESS CHECK (Did I have any sick days?):

_____

_____

BODY WEIGHT: MONTHLY CYCLE DATES (if applicable):

_____

DOCTOR/DENTIST APPOINTMENTS:

Teeth Cleaned (Jan)

MEDICATIONS TAKEN:

_____

Taking Small Steps
(The Power of Progression)

G rowing up, I hated flossing my teeth. Then my dentist put in me the fear of losing them if I didn't start flossing every day. I knew I couldn't do that, so I put a container of new floss on the counter and told myself to floss once a week as a start. I felt I could handle that much. Gradually, I added more days of flossing each week, until I made it a daily habit. And today I have very good teeth!

Little did I know when I was younger that I was laying the groundwork for later promoting exercise and eating well with guidance that proves out every time: Permanent change happens when the change is initiated with small steps. Many people feel they have to go from 0 to 100 in 10 seconds flat—which usually leads to disastrous results. They burn out quickly, injure themselves, end up bingeing—or engaging in any range of unhealthy behaviors.

That's why, if your aim is to become more physically active and you are now completely sedentary, you will find success by starting slowly and walking 10 minutes three times a week and doing two or three strength-training exercises once a week. After 2 to 4 weeks, you can reevaluate, seeing whether you have enough energy to increase your distance or pace or exercises in your strength-training sessions.

It's the same with food. You can't turn around your entire diet in a day. What I often tell people who want to start eating better—either for weight loss or all-around health—is to begin by making sure they eat three servings of vegetables every day and taking it from there. It's more manageable than tackling sweets and other categories all at once. Over time, one good move motivates people to try another, until a clear rhythm emerges and the pounds start coming off. *That's* the power of progression.

February

FEBRUARY 1–7

Ten years ago I injured my back. I assumed the injury would go away, but it didn't. Over the course of a year, I stopped exercising. In fact, I became afraid of it. One day my husband wanted to teach me how to cross-country ski. I was so nervous about my back that I was shaking. But I did it. And when I got home, I found that my back felt better. It was a light bulb going off: Strength begets strength.—MOLLY

PERSONAL NOTES

FEBRUARY 1, DAY OF THE WEEK   S   M   T   W   TH   F   S

MOOD	VIGOR	SLEEP
Excellent		
□	□	□
□	□	□
□	□	□
Poor		

FEBRUARY 2, DAY OF THE WEEK   S   M   T   W   TH   F   S

MOOD	VIGOR	SLEEP
Excellent		
□	□	□
□	□	□
□	□	□
Poor		

FEBRUARY 3, DAY OF THE WEEK   S   M   T   W   TH   F   S

MOOD	VIGOR	SLEEP
Excellent		
□	□	□
□	□	□
□	□	□
Poor		

Many women fear breast cancer more than any other illness, but heart disease is women's number-one cause of death. Breast cancer kills about 45,000 women a year; heart disease, half a million. That's why it's so important to eat right and exercise regularly. A healthful lifestyle is the first line of defense against cardiovascular problems.

FEBRUARY 4, DAY OF THE WEEK S M T W TH F S

MOOD	VIGOR	SLEEP
Excellent		
☐	☐	☐
☐	☐	☐
☐	☐	☐
Poor		

FEBRUARY 5, DAY OF THE WEEK S M T W TH F S

MOOD	VIGOR	SLEEP
Excellent		
☐	☐	☐
☐	☐	☐
☐	☐	☐
Poor		

FEBRUARY 6, DAY OF THE WEEK S M T W TH F S

MOOD	VIGOR	SLEEP
Excellent		
☐	☐	☐
☐	☐	☐
☐	☐	☐
Poor		

FEBRUARY 7, DAY OF THE WEEK S M T W TH F S

MOOD	VIGOR	SLEEP
Excellent		
☐	☐	☐
☐	☐	☐
☐	☐	☐
Poor		

FEBRUARY 1–7
NUTRITION LOG

GOALS (# SERVINGS)	WHOLE GRAINS 3+	FRUITS 2+	VEGETABLES 3+	PROTEIN 2–4	DAIRY 2–3	EXTRAS VARIABLE
FEBRUARY 1	☐	☐	☐	☐	☐	☐
NOTES:						
FEBRUARY 2	☐	☐	☐	☐	☐	☐
NOTES:						
FEBRUARY 3	☐	☐	☐	☐	☐	☐
NOTES:						
FEBRUARY 4	☐	☐	☐	☐	☐	☐
NOTES:						
FEBRUARY 5	☐	☐	☐	☐	☐	☐
NOTES:						
FEBRUARY 6	☐	☐	☐	☐	☐	☐
NOTES:						
FEBRUARY 7	☐	☐	☐	☐	☐	☐
NOTES:						

CALCIUM + VITAMIN D ☐ VITAMIN E ☐ MULTIVITAMIN/MINERAL ☐

PLENTY OF FLUIDS ☐ OTHER SUPPLEMENTS _____

OVERALL COMMENTS

PHYSICAL ACTIVITY

planned, sport, leisure, errands, play
Goal: 30 to 60 minutes most days of the week

DAY	ACTIVITY	TIME

STRENGTH TRAINING

Goal: 2 to 3 times per week

EXERCISE 2 SETS/8 TO 10 REPS	DAY: POUNDS OR ✓	DAY: POUNDS OR ✓	DAY: POUNDS OR ✓

NUMBER OF STEPS

FEBRUARY 1   FEBRUARY 2   FEBRUARY 3   FEBRUARY 4   FEBRUARY 5   FEBRUARY 6   FEBRUARY 7

_____   _____   _____   _____   _____   _____   _____

FEBRUARY 8–14

I have come to realize that the ability to change what you don't like is remarkable. But the discretion to know when to use that ability is all the more impressive. I can try to change the body I was given. I can starve, obsessively work out, and schedule liposuction to achieve a certain standard. Thankfully, my discretion tells me to continue eating healthy, work out sensibly, and achieve the balance that keeps me stronger than ever.—ERICA

PERSONAL NOTES

FEBRUARY 8, DAY OF THE WEEK   S   M   T   W   TH   F   S

MOOD	VIGOR	SLEEP
	Excellent	
☐	☐	☐
☐	☐	☐
☐	☐	☐
	Poor	

FEBRUARY 9, DAY OF THE WEEK   S   M   T   W   TH   F   S

MOOD	VIGOR	SLEEP
	Excellent	
☐	☐	☐
☐	☐	☐
☐	☐	☐
	Poor	

FEBRUARY 10, DAY OF THE WEEK   S   M   T   W   TH   F   S

MOOD	VIGOR	SLEEP
	Excellent	
☐	☐	☐
☐	☐	☐
☐	☐	☐
	Poor	

Try a Japanese restaurant when you want to eat out. Restaurants these days serve gargantuan portions with lots of calories and fat, but Japanese restaurants have some pretty reasonable choices. For instance, an entrée called Nabeyaki-Udon—thick noodles served in a light fish broth with shrimp, vegetables, and an egg—contains just 510 calories, according to an analysis of Japanese food conducted by the *Tufts University Health & Nutrition Letter*. Six pieces of Tekka Maki sushi—rice and raw tuna—provide only about 170 calories.

FEBRUARY 11, DAY OF THE WEEK   S   M   T   W   TH   F   S

MOOD	VIGOR	SLEEP
Excellent		
☐	☐	☐
☐	☐	☐
☐	☐	☐
Poor		

FEBRUARY 12, DAY OF THE WEEK   S   M   T   W   TH   F   S

MOOD	VIGOR	SLEEP
Excellent		
☐	☐	☐
☐	☐	☐
☐	☐	☐
Poor		

FEBRUARY 13, DAY OF THE WEEK   S   M   T   W   TH   F   S

MOOD	VIGOR	SLEEP
Excellent		
☐	☐	☐
☐	☐	☐
☐	☐	☐
Poor		

FEBRUARY 14, DAY OF THE WEEK   S   M   T   W   TH   F   S

MOOD	VIGOR	SLEEP
Excellent		
☐	☐	☐
☐	☐	☐
☐	☐	☐
Poor		

FEBRUARY 8–14
NUTRITION LOG

GOALS (# SERVINGS)	WHOLE GRAINS 3+	FRUITS 2+	VEGETABLES 3+	PROTEIN 2–4	DAIRY 2–3	EXTRAS VARIABLE
FEBRUARY 8 NOTES:	☐	☐	☐	☐	☐	☐
FEBRUARY 9 NOTES:	☐	☐	☐	☐	☐	☐
FEBRUARY 10 NOTES:	☐	☐	☐	☐	☐	☐
FEBRUARY 11 NOTES:	☐	☐	☐	☐	☐	☐
FEBRUARY 12 NOTES:	☐	☐	☐	☐	☐	☐
FEBRUARY 13 NOTES:	☐	☐	☐	☐	☐	☐
FEBRUARY 14 NOTES:	☐	☐	☐	☐	☐	☐

CALCIUM + VITAMIN D ☐ VITAMIN E ☐ MULTIVITAMIN/MINERAL ☐

PLENTY OF FLUIDS ☐ OTHER SUPPLEMENTS _____

OVERALL COMMENTS

PHYSICAL ACTIVITY

planned, sport, leisure, errands, play
Goal: 30 to 60 minutes most days of the week

DAY	ACTIVITY	TIME

STRENGTH TRAINING

Goal: 2 to 3 times per week

EXERCISE 2 SETS/8 TO 10 REPS	DAY: POUNDS OR ✓	DAY: POUNDS OR ✓	DAY: POUNDS OR ✓

NUMBER OF STEPS

FEBRUARY 8 FEBRUARY 9 FEBRUARY 10 FEBRUARY 11 FEBRUARY 12 FEBRUARY 13 FEBRUARY 14

FEBRUARY 15–21

The week I began my radiation treatment for cancer at age 39, my brother was killed by a drunk driver. I was suddenly living alone in the two-family home we shared, devastated physically and emotionally. I had no choice but to move forward, so I decided to do it with strength, purpose, and as much grace as I could muster. I began with my physical strength. A solo trip to a health spa inspired me to begin a program of healthy eating, weight lifting, and yoga that I've maintained for the past 3 years. For my inner strength, I began a foundation in my brother's name to benefit local Little League alumni. I recently turned to my personal life—having a past marriage annulled and taking back my maiden name. This is all new to me, but I know that every step forward is bringing me to where I'm meant to be. I feel the strongest I have ever felt, physically and emotionally, and life is good.—BETH

PERSONAL NOTES

FEBRUARY 15, DAY OF THE WEEK   S   M   T   W   TH   F   S

MOOD	VIGOR	SLEEP
	Excellent	
☐	☐	☐
☐	☐	☐
☐	☐	☐
	Poor	

FEBRUARY 16, DAY OF THE WEEK   S   M   T   W   TH   F   S

MOOD	VIGOR	SLEEP
	Excellent	
☐	☐	☐
☐	☐	☐
☐	☐	☐
	Poor	

FEBRUARY 17, DAY OF THE WEEK   S   M   T   W   TH   F   S

MOOD	VIGOR	SLEEP
	Excellent	
☐	☐	☐
☐	☐	☐
☐	☐	☐
	Poor	

A personal trainer can be expensive—up to $120 an hour, depending on where you live. But you can go in with some friends on several sessions with a trainer to keep down the cost. A personal trainer can really help with the finer points of strength training so that you 1) target your muscles correctly during each exercise in order to achieve maximum gain; 2) avoid injury as you lift or pull; and 3) choose the moves that are most likely to give you the outcomes in strength and body toning that you desire.

FEBRUARY 18, DAY OF THE WEEK   S   M   T   W   TH   F   S

MOOD	VIGOR	SLEEP
Excellent		
☐	☐	☐
☐	☐	☐
☐	☐	☐
Poor		

FEBRUARY 19, DAY OF THE WEEK   S   M   T   W   TH   F   S

MOOD	VIGOR	SLEEP
Excellent		
☐	☐	☐
☐	☐	☐
☐	☐	☐
Poor		

FEBRUARY 20, DAY OF THE WEEK   S   M   T   W   TH   F   S

MOOD	VIGOR	SLEEP
Excellent		
☐	☐	☐
☐	☐	☐
☐	☐	☐
Poor		

FEBRUARY 21, DAY OF THE WEEK   S   M   T   W   TH   F   S

MOOD	VIGOR	SLEEP
Excellent		
☐	☐	☐
☐	☐	☐
☐	☐	☐
Poor		

FEBRUARY 15–21
NUTRITION LOG

GOALS (# SERVINGS)	WHOLE GRAINS	FRUITS	VEGETABLES	PROTEIN	DAIRY	EXTRAS
	3+	2+	3+	2–4	2–3	VARIABLE
FEBRUARY 15	☐	☐	☐	☐	☐	☐
NOTES:						
FEBRUARY 16	☐	☐	☐	☐	☐	☐
NOTES:						
FEBRUARY 17	☐	☐	☐	☐	☐	☐
NOTES:						
FEBRUARY 18	☐	☐	☐	☐	☐	☐
NOTES:						
FEBRUARY 19	☐	☐	☐	☐	☐	☐
NOTES:						
FEBRUARY 20	☐	☐	☐	☐	☐	☐
NOTES:						
FEBRUARY 21	☐	☐	☐	☐	☐	☐
NOTES:						

CALCIUM + VITAMIN D ☐ VITAMIN E ☐ MULTIVITAMIN/MINERAL ☐

PLENTY OF FLUIDS ☐ OTHER SUPPLEMENTS _____

OVERALL COMMENTS

PHYSICAL ACTIVITY

planned, sport, leisure, errands, play
Goal: 30 to 60 minutes most days of the week

DAY	ACTIVITY	TIME

STRENGTH TRAINING

Goal: 2 to 3 times per week

EXERCISE 2 SETS/8 TO 10 REPS	DAY: POUNDS OR ✓	DAY: POUNDS OR ✓	DAY: POUNDS OR ✓

NUMBER OF STEPS

FEBRUARY 15   FEBRUARY 16   FEBRUARY 17   FEBRUARY 18   FEBRUARY 19   FEBRUARY 20   FEBRUARY 21

FEBRUARY 22–28

*In the past year, I have become a new woman: I can run longer and faster, I joined a women's soccer team, I've tried countless new recipes. How did I do all this? I have eliminated the things in my life that discouraged me. Instead of always meeting at a bar or restaurant, I drag friends to the gym or to the park to exercise. I've found new magazines with a positive focus on wellness and have eliminated the ones that promote unrealistic beauty ideals and use super-skinny models. I have discovered an online community of women devoted to healthy weight loss. Most importantly, I avoid guilt and desperation at all costs by occasionally indulging in foods I love.—*REBECCA

PERSONAL NOTES

FEBRUARY 22, DAY OF THE WEEK   S   M   T   W   TH   F   S

MOOD	VIGOR	SLEEP
Excellent		
☐	☐	☐
☐	☐	☐
☐	☐	☐
Poor		

FEBRUARY 23, DAY OF THE WEEK   S   M   T   W   TH   F   S

MOOD	VIGOR	SLEEP
Excellent		
☐	☐	☐
☐	☐	☐
☐	☐	☐
Poor		

FEBRUARY 24, DAY OF THE WEEK   S   M   T   W   TH   F   S

MOOD	VIGOR	SLEEP
Excellent		
☐	☐	☐
☐	☐	☐
☐	☐	☐
Poor		

Cereal rules! It's an easy, healthful breakfast—one of the top sources of folate, iron, and vitamin B_6 in the U.S. diet. Good cereal rules to follow: at least three grams of fiber per serving; no more than 3 to 5 grams of sugar (about a teaspoon's worth); and no more than 200 milligrams of sodium. Check the Nutrition Facts panel on the side of the box.

FEBRUARY 25, DAY OF THE WEEK   S   M   T   W   TH   F   S

MOOD	VIGOR	SLEEP
Excellent		
☐	☐	☐
☐	☐	☐
☐	☐	☐
Poor		

FEBRUARY 26, DAY OF THE WEEK   S   M   T   W   TH   F   S

MOOD	VIGOR	SLEEP
Excellent		
☐	☐	☐
☐	☐	☐
☐	☐	☐
Poor		

FEBRUARY 27, DAY OF THE WEEK   S   M   T   W   TH   F   S

MOOD	VIGOR	SLEEP
Excellent		
☐	☐	☐
☐	☐	☐
☐	☐	☐
Poor		

FEBRUARY 28, DAY OF THE WEEK   S   M   T   W   TH   F   S

MOOD	VIGOR	SLEEP
Excellent		
☐	☐	☐
☐	☐	☐
☐	☐	☐
Poor		

FEBRUARY 22–28
NUTRITION LOG

GOALS (# SERVINGS)	WHOLE GRAINS 3+	FRUITS 2+	VEGETABLES 3+	PROTEIN 2–4	DAIRY 2–3	EXTRAS VARIABLE
FEBRUARY 22 NOTES:	☐	☐	☐	☐	☐	☐
FEBRUARY 23 NOTES:	☐	☐	☐	☐	☐	☐
FEBRUARY 24 NOTES:	☐	☐	☐	☐	☐	☐
FEBRUARY 25 NOTES:	☐	☐	☐	☐	☐	☐
FEBRUARY 26 NOTES:	☐	☐	☐	☐	☐	☐
FEBRUARY 27 NOTES:	☐	☐	☐	☐	☐	☐
FEBRUARY 28 NOTES:	☐	☐	☐	☐	☐	☐

CALCIUM + VITAMIN D ☐ VITAMIN E ☐ MULTIVITAMIN/MINERAL ☐

PLENTY OF FLUIDS ☐ OTHER SUPPLEMENTS _____

OVERALL COMMENTS

PHYSICAL ACTIVITY

planned, sport, leisure, errands, play
Goal: 30 to 60 minutes most days of the week

DAY	ACTIVITY	TIME

STRENGTH TRAINING

Goal: 2 to 3 times per week

EXERCISE 2 SETS/8 TO 10 REPS	DAY: POUNDS OR ✓	DAY: POUNDS OR ✓	DAY: POUNDS OR ✓

NUMBER OF STEPS

FEBRUARY 22	FEBRUARY 23	FEBRUARY 24	FEBRUARY 25	FEBRUARY 26	FEBRUARY 27	FEBRUARY 28

FEBRUARY 29

I'm 54, and the only exercise that I truly like is gardening. I love to really dig, and double-dig, all of my flower and vegetable beds. But during non-digging months (i.e., October–April), I get very little exercise and usually have lots of aches and pains in late spring. Last spring I started doing weight training for the first time and I had no aches at all. In fact, I had no pain in the knee that I had injured 20+ years ago. (Usually that knee has plagued me during gardening season.) But the topper is this: I've had a snow blower for 18 years and have always needed to find testosterone-filled muscles to start the thing. Last week, in preparation for the first snowstorm of the season, I started that machine on the very first try! I can't tell you what it means to be strong enough to do that!—ROSELLEN

PERSONAL NOTES

FEBRUARY 29, DAY OF THE WEEK S M T W TH F S

	MOOD	VIGOR	SLEEP
Excellent			
	☐	☐	☐
	☐	☐	☐
	☐	☐	☐
Poor			

NUTRITION LOG

	WHOLE GRAINS	FRUITS	VEGETABLES	PROTEIN	DAIRY	EXTRAS
GOALS (# SERVINGS)	3+	2+	3+	2–4	2–3	VARIABLE
FEBRUARY 29	☐	☐	☐	☐	☐	☐

NOTES:

CALCIUM + VITAMIN D ☐ VITAMIN E ☐ MULTIVITAMIN/MINERAL ☐

PLENTY OF FLUIDS ☐ OTHER SUPPLEMENTS _____

OVERALL COMMENTS

PHYSICAL ACTIVITY

planned, sport, leisure, errands, play
Goal: 30 to 60 minutes most days of the week

DAY	ACTIVITY	TIME

STRENGTH TRAINING

Goal: 2 to 3 times per week

EXERCISE 2 SETS/8 TO 10 REPS	DAY: POUNDS OR ✓	DAY: POUNDS OR ✓	DAY: POUNDS OR ✓

NUMBER OF STEPS

FEBRUARY 29

FEBRUARY REVIEW

BRIGHT SPOTS:

_____

GREATEST CHALLENGES:

_____

_____

PATTERNS OBSERVED:

_____

IDENTIFY BARRIERS TO CHANGE AND HOW I AM GOING TO OVERCOME THEM:

    PERSONAL

_____

_____

    PROFESSIONAL

_____

_____

PERSONAL CARE ATTENTION (flossing teeth, skin care, cutting/coloring hair, etc.):

_____

_____

WELLNESS CHECK (Did I have any sick days?):

_____

_____

BODY WEIGHT: MONTHLY CYCLE DATES (if applicable):

_____

DOCTOR/DENTIST APPOINTMENTS:

_____

_____

MEDICATIONS TAKEN:

_____

_____

_____

A Leap of Faith
(Trying Something Before It Feels Comfortable)

~᭞᭞~

I have always been afraid of heights, and everyone who knows me is aware of this. So when my friend, Kristin, and her husband tried to get me to go rock climbing with them one day, I told them they were crazy. But they cajoled me until I gave in. At first I was really bad at my attempts to scamper up the cliffs. Although I was safely attached to Kristin via a rope, I was scared half to death of being up so high. Now, five years later, my whole family rock climbs. I still get frightened sometimes. But, I love it and am proud of my accomplishment—even if my children are better at it than me!

The point is that it's always easier to try something once you feel ready, but for some things you can wait a lifetime to feel ready and miss your chance. There are times you have to try things *before* they feel right.

This is particularly true with exercise. Many woman don't want to start because exercising exhausts them, and they feel tired in the first place. But within six weeks, exercising actually makes people more energetic than they were before.

Strength-training gains come even sooner. Mary, a woman in her 50s who wrote to me from England, exemplifies the point beautifully. After having been sedentary for many years, she finally took the leap.

"I have been doing your *Strong Women Stay Slim* program for just two weeks every other day," she wrote. "I have already progressed from one pound to two pounds on the overhead press, bent-over row, and arm curl. Within two to three days I felt more confident and more full of desire for my husband. I definitely have more energy for gardening and so forth. And after decades of hiding my flabby upper arms, my arms feel firmer."

Don't wait decades. Take your leap today!

March

MARCH 1–7

Five months ago, I began the journey toward becoming healthy again. I had, unbelievably, gained 56 pounds over 5 years and was overwhelmed by the task ahead. I have now lost 26 pounds and really feel I am strong enough to go all the way. My secret for staying strong physically and emotionally is setting my alarm for 6 A.M. and going for my walk at the break of dawn. I have only 30 minutes before I have to get ready for work, but those 30 minutes make all the difference in my day.—KAREN

PERSONAL NOTES

MARCH 1, DAY OF THE WEEK   S   M   T   W   TH   F   S

MOOD	VIGOR	SLEEP
Excellent		
☐	☐	☐
☐	☐	☐
☐	☐	☐
Poor		

MARCH 2, DAY OF THE WEEK   S   M   T   W   TH   F   S

MOOD	VIGOR	SLEEP
Excellent		
☐	☐	☐
☐	☐	☐
☐	☐	☐
Poor		

MARCH 3, DAY OF THE WEEK   S   M   T   W   TH   F   S

MOOD	VIGOR	SLEEP
Excellent		
☐	☐	☐
☐	☐	☐
☐	☐	☐
Poor		

Do some upper body stretches for three to five minutes out of every hour that you are sitting at a desk. For example, tip your head left, right, and forward, and pull back your shoulder blades. It will relax you as well as promote flexibility.

MARCH 4, DAY OF THE WEEK   S   M   T   W   TH   F   S

MOOD	VIGOR	SLEEP
Excellent		
☐	☐	☐
☐	☐	☐
☐	☐	☐
Poor		

MARCH 5, DAY OF THE WEEK   S   M   T   W   TH   F   S

MOOD	VIGOR	SLEEP
Excellent		
☐	☐	☐
☐	☐	☐
☐	☐	☐
Poor		

MARCH 6, DAY OF THE WEEK   S   M   T   W   TH   F   S

MOOD	VIGOR	SLEEP
Excellent		
☐	☐	☐
☐	☐	☐
☐	☐	☐
Poor		

MARCH 7, DAY OF THE WEEK   S   M   T   W   TH   F   S

MOOD	VIGOR	SLEEP
Excellent		
☐	☐	☐
☐	☐	☐
☐	☐	☐
Poor		

MARCH 1–7
NUTRITION LOG

GOALS (# SERVINGS)	WHOLE GRAINS 3+	FRUITS 2+	VEGETABLES 3+	PROTEIN 2–4	DAIRY 2–3	EXTRAS VARIABLE
MARCH 1	☐	☐	☐	☐	☐	☐
NOTES:						
MARCH 2	☐	☐	☐	☐	☐	☐
NOTES:						
MARCH 3	☐	☐	☐	☐	☐	☐
NOTES:						
MARCH 4	☐	☐	☐	☐	☐	☐
NOTES:						
MARCH 5	☐	☐	☐	☐	☐	☐
NOTES:						
MARCH 6	☐	☐	☐	☐	☐	☐
NOTES:						
MARCH 7	☐	☐	☐	☐	☐	☐
NOTES:						

CALCIUM + VITAMIN D ☐ **VITAMIN E** ☐ **MULTIVITAMIN/MINERAL** ☐

PLENTY OF FLUIDS ☐ **OTHER SUPPLEMENTS** _____

OVERALL COMMENTS

PHYSICAL ACTIVITY

planned, sport, leisure, errands, play
Goal: 30 to 60 minutes most days of the week

DAY	ACTIVITY	TIME

STRENGTH TRAINING

Goal: 2 to 3 times per week

EXERCISE 2 SETS/8 TO 10 REPS	DAY: POUNDS OR ✓	DAY: POUNDS OR ✓	DAY: POUNDS OR ✓

NUMBER OF STEPS

MARCH 1	MARCH 2	MARCH 3	MARCH 4	MARCH 5	MARCH 6	MARCH 7

MARCH 8–14

Being a recently divorced mother of three, a self-employed research consultant, and a full-time Ph.D. student, maintaining my physical and emotional health can be quite challenging. Like most women, I have spent a lot of time sacrificing my own well-being for that of others in my life. However, one day as I was sitting at my children's Tae Kwon Do class, I had an inspiration. I was going to take advantage of the family discount and start doing the class with them. Practicing martial arts has improved my mental well-being by taking me away from the stresses in my life. Additionally, I have increased my physical strength and endurance. I now work out regularly, both with and without my children, and feel stronger than ever before. The secret is finding an activity that fits smoothly with what you are already doing.—MARY

PERSONAL NOTES

MARCH 8, DAY OF THE WEEK   S   M   T   W   TH   F   S

MOOD	VIGOR	SLEEP
Excellent		
☐	☐	☐
☐	☐	☐
☐	☐	☐
Poor		

MARCH 9, DAY OF THE WEEK   S   M   T   W   TH   F   S

MOOD	VIGOR	SLEEP
Excellent		
☐	☐	☐
☐	☐	☐
☐	☐	☐
Poor		

MARCH 10, DAY OF THE WEEK   S   M   T   W   TH   F   S

MOOD	VIGOR	SLEEP
Excellent		
☐	☐	☐
☐	☐	☐
☐	☐	☐
Poor		

Vegetable-topped pizza tends to mean pizza flecked with a few bits of pepper or broccoli. When ordering in, heat up a package of frozen broccoli or spinach, and spoon a half-cup over a slice or two. That way, you won't lose out on any of the cheesy, spicy flavor, but your dinner will *really* come with one out of the three to five servings of vegetables you're supposed to have every day.

MARCH 11, DAY OF THE WEEK   S   M   T   W   TH   F   S

MOOD	VIGOR	SLEEP
Excellent		
☐	☐	☐
☐	☐	☐
☐	☐	☐
Poor		

MARCH 12, DAY OF THE WEEK   S   M   T   W   TH   F   S

MOOD	VIGOR	SLEEP
Excellent		
☐	☐	☐
☐	☐	☐
☐	☐	☐
Poor		

MARCH 13, DAY OF THE WEEK   S   M   T   W   TH   F   S

MOOD	VIGOR	SLEEP
Excellent		
☐	☐	☐
☐	☐	☐
☐	☐	☐
Poor		

MARCH 14, DAY OF THE WEEK   S   M   T   W   TH   F   S

MOOD	VIGOR	SLEEP
Excellent		
☐	☐	☐
☐	☐	☐
☐	☐	☐
Poor		

MARCH 8–14
NUTRITION LOG

GOALS (# SERVINGS)	WHOLE GRAINS 3+	FRUITS 2+	VEGETABLES 3+	PROTEIN 2–4	DAIRY 2–3	EXTRAS VARIABLE
MARCH 8 NOTES:	☐	☐	☐	☐	☐	☐
MARCH 9 NOTES:	☐	☐	☐	☐	☐	☐
MARCH 10 NOTES:	☐	☐	☐	☐	☐	☐
MARCH 11 NOTES:	☐	☐	☐	☐	☐	☐
MARCH 12 NOTES:	☐	☐	☐	☐	☐	☐
MARCH 13 NOTES:	☐	☐	☐	☐	☐	☐
MARCH 14 NOTES:	☐	☐	☐	☐	☐	☐

CALCIUM + VITAMIN D ☐ VITAMIN E ☐ MULTIVITAMIN/MINERAL ☐

PLENTY OF FLUIDS ☐ OTHER SUPPLEMENTS _____

OVERALL COMMENTS

PHYSICAL ACTIVITY

planned, sport, leisure, errands, play
Goal: 30 to 60 minutes most days of the week

DAY	ACTIVITY	TIME

STRENGTH TRAINING

Goal: 2 to 3 times per week

EXERCISE 2 SETS/8 TO 10 REPS	DAY: POUNDS OR ✓	DAY: POUNDS OR ✓	DAY: POUNDS OR ✓

NUMBER OF STEPS

MARCH 8	MARCH 9	MARCH 10	MARCH 11	MARCH 12	MARCH 13	MARCH 14

MARCH 15–21

I've been exercising in the morning, right after I brush my teeth, for the last 16 years. That way, when problems come up later that mean I have to stay late at the office—or if I decide at the last minute to go out with friends—I haven't missed a workout.—LAURA

PERSONAL NOTES

MARCH 15, DAY OF THE WEEK S M T W TH F S

MOOD	VIGOR	SLEEP
	Excellent	
☐	☐	☐
☐	☐	☐
☐	☐	☐
	Poor	

MARCH 16, DAY OF THE WEEK S M T W TH F S

MOOD	VIGOR	SLEEP
	Excellent	
☐	☐	☐
☐	☐	☐
☐	☐	☐
	Poor	

MARCH 17, DAY OF THE WEEK S M T W TH F S

MOOD	VIGOR	SLEEP
	Excellent	
☐	☐	☐
☐	☐	☐
☐	☐	☐
	Poor	

While stretching after exercise is crucial for keeping your muscles, tendons, and ligaments flexible, you don't necessarily need to stretch *before* exercising. You should, however, warm up just prior to working out. For aerobics, that means doing the aerobic exercise at a slower pace than you plan to for the duration of your workout. For strength training, it means lifting less weight than you normally would for a few reps. Moving around or lifting with "cold," unprepared muscles can cause unnecessary strains and tears in muscle tissue.

MARCH 18, DAY OF THE WEEK S M T W TH F S

MOOD	VIGOR	SLEEP
Excellent		
□	□	□
□	□	□
□	□	□
Poor		

MARCH 19, DAY OF THE WEEK S M T W TH F S

MOOD	VIGOR	SLEEP
Excellent		
□	□	□
□	□	□
□	□	□
Poor		

MARCH 20, DAY OF THE WEEK S M T W TH F S

MOOD	VIGOR	SLEEP
Excellent		
□	□	□
□	□	□
□	□	□
Poor		

MARCH 21, DAY OF THE WEEK S M T W TH F S

MOOD	VIGOR	SLEEP
Excellent		
□	□	□
□	□	□
□	□	□
Poor		

MARCH 15–21
NUTRITION LOG

GOALS (# SERVINGS)	WHOLE GRAINS 3+	FRUITS 2+	VEGETABLES 3+	PROTEIN 2–4	DAIRY 2–3	EXTRAS VARIABLE
MARCH 15 **NOTES:**	☐	☐	☐	☐	☐	☐
MARCH 16 **NOTES:**	☐	☐	☐	☐	☐	☐
MARCH 17 **NOTES:**	☐	☐	☐	☐	☐	☐
MARCH 18 **NOTES:**	☐	☐	☐	☐	☐	☐
MARCH 19 **NOTES:**	☐	☐	☐	☐	☐	☐
MARCH 20 **NOTES:**	☐	☐	☐	☐	☐	☐
MARCH 21 **NOTES:**	☐	☐	☐	☐	☐	☐

CALCIUM + VITAMIN D ☐ **VITAMIN E** ☐ **MULTIVITAMIN/MINERAL** ☐

PLENTY OF FLUIDS ☐ **OTHER SUPPLEMENTS** _____

OVERALL COMMENTS

PHYSICAL ACTIVITY

planned, sport, leisure, errands, play
Goal: 30 to 60 minutes most days of the week

DAY	ACTIVITY	TIME

STRENGTH TRAINING

Goal: 2 to 3 times per week

EXERCISE 2 SETS/8 TO 10 REPS	DAY: POUNDS OR ✓	DAY: POUNDS OR ✓	DAY: POUNDS OR ✓

NUMBER OF STEPS

MARCH 15   MARCH 16   MARCH 17   MARCH 18   MARCH 19   MARCH 20   MARCH 21

_____   _____   _____   _____   _____   _____   _____

MARCH 22–28

As a radio personality, I'm alone in the studio for hours at a time. I bring my dumbbells to work and use them while I play long songs. I do lunges, squats, and any other exercise that I can think of. Every little bit helps.—HOLLIS

PERSONAL NOTES

MARCH 22, DAY OF THE WEEK   S   M   T   W   TH   F   S

MOOD	VIGOR	SLEEP
Excellent		
☐	☐	☐
☐	☐	☐
☐	☐	☐
Poor		

MARCH 23, DAY OF THE WEEK   S   M   T   W   TH   F   S

MOOD	VIGOR	SLEEP
Excellent		
☐	☐	☐
☐	☐	☐
☐	☐	☐
Poor		

MARCH 24, DAY OF THE WEEK   S   M   T   W   TH   F   S

MOOD	VIGOR	SLEEP
Excellent		
☐	☐	☐
☐	☐	☐
☐	☐	☐
Poor		

For an easy, healthful salsa on grilled fish or chicken, mix tropical fruit cocktail with chopped onion, a dash of cilantro, and a splash of lemon juice.

MARCH 25, DAY OF THE WEEK   S   M   T   W   TH   F   S

	MOOD	VIGOR	SLEEP
	Excellent		
	☐	☐	☐
	☐	☐	☐
	☐	☐	☐
	Poor		

MARCH 26, DAY OF THE WEEK   S   M   T   W   TH   F   S

	MOOD	VIGOR	SLEEP
	Excellent		
	☐	☐	☐
	☐	☐	☐
	☐	☐	☐
	Poor		

MARCH 27, DAY OF THE WEEK   S   M   T   W   TH   F   S

	MOOD	VIGOR	SLEEP
	Excellent		
	☐	☐	☐
	☐	☐	☐
	☐	☐	☐
	Poor		

MARCH 28, DAY OF THE WEEK   S   M   T   W   TH   F   S

	MOOD	VIGOR	SLEEP
	Excellent		
	☐	☐	☐
	☐	☐	☐
	☐	☐	☐
	Poor		

MARCH 22–28
NUTRITION LOG

GOALS (# SERVINGS)	WHOLE GRAINS 3+	FRUITS 2+	VEGETABLES 3+	PROTEIN 2–4	DAIRY 2–3	EXTRAS VARIABLE
MARCH 22 NOTES:	☐	☐	☐	☐	☐	☐
MARCH 23 NOTES:	☐	☐	☐	☐	☐	☐
MARCH 24 NOTES:	☐	☐	☐	☐	☐	☐
MARCH 25 NOTES:	☐	☐	☐	☐	☐	☐
MARCH 26 NOTES:	☐	☐	☐	☐	☐	☐
MARCH 27 NOTES:	☐	☐	☐	☐	☐	☐
MARCH 28 NOTES:	☐	☐	☐	☐	☐	☐

CALCIUM + VITAMIN D ☐ **VITAMIN E** ☐ **MULTIVITAMIN/MINERAL** ☐

PLENTY OF FLUIDS ☐ **OTHER SUPPLEMENTS** _____

OVERALL COMMENTS

PHYSICAL ACTIVITY

planned, sport, leisure, errands, play
Goal: 30 to 60 minutes most days of the week

DAY	ACTIVITY	TIME

STRENGTH TRAINING

Goal: 2 to 3 times per week

EXERCISE 2 SETS/8 TO 10 REPS	DAY: POUNDS OR ✓	DAY: POUNDS OR ✓	DAY: POUNDS OR ✓

NUMBER OF STEPS

MARCH 22	MARCH 23	MARCH 24	MARCH 25	MARCH 26	MARCH 27	MARCH 28

MARCH 29–31

PERSONAL NOTES

MARCH 29, DAY OF THE WEEK   S   M   T   W   TH   F   S

MOOD	VIGOR	SLEEP
	Excellent	
☐	☐	☐
☐	☐	☐
☐	☐	☐
	Poor	

MARCH 30, DAY OF THE WEEK   S   M   T   W   TH   F   S

MOOD	VIGOR	SLEEP
	Excellent	
☐	☐	☐
☐	☐	☐
☐	☐	☐
	Poor	

MARCH 31, DAY OF THE WEEK   S   M   T   W   TH   F   S

MOOD	VIGOR	SLEEP
	Excellent	
☐	☐	☐
☐	☐	☐
☐	☐	☐
	Poor	

March 29–31
Nutrition Log

	WHOLE GRAINS	FRUITS	VEGETABLES	PROTEIN	DAIRY	EXTRAS
GOALS (# SERVINGS)	3+	2+	3+	2–4	2–3	VARIABLE
MARCH 29	☐	☐	☐	☐	☐	☐

NOTES:

MARCH 30	☐	☐	☐	☐	☐	☐

NOTES:

MARCH 31	☐	☐	☐	☐	☐	☐

NOTES:

CALCIUM + VITAMIN D ☐   VITAMIN E ☐   MULTIVITAMIN/MINERAL ☐

PLENTY OF FLUIDS ☐   OTHER SUPPLEMENTS _____

OVERALL COMMENTS

PHYSICAL ACTIVITY

planned, sport, leisure, errands, play
Goal: 30 to 60 minutes most days of the week

DAY	ACTIVITY	TIME

STRENGTH TRAINING

Goal: 2 to 3 times per week

EXERCISE 2 SETS/8 TO 10 REPS	DAY: POUNDS OR ✓	DAY: POUNDS OR ✓	DAY: POUNDS OR ✓

NUMBER OF STEPS

MARCH 29   MARCH 30   MARCH 31

_____   _____   _____

MARCH REVIEW

BRIGHT SPOTS:
_____
_____

GREATEST CHALLENGES:
_____
_____
_____

PATTERNS OBSERVED:
_____
_____

IDENTIFY BARRIERS TO CHANGE AND HOW I AM GOING TO OVERCOME THEM:

PERSONAL
_____
_____
_____

PROFESSIONAL
_____
_____
_____

PERSONAL CARE ATTENTION (flossing teeth, skin care, cutting/coloring hair, etc.):
_____
_____
_____

WELLNESS CHECK (Did I have any sick days?):
_____
_____
_____

BODY WEIGHT: MONTHLY CYCLE DATES (if applicable):
_____
_____

DOCTOR/DENTIST APPOINTMENTS:
_____
_____
_____

MEDICATIONS TAKEN:
_____
_____
_____

I Don't Have Time

෴

"Once I understood that the world was not going to carve out the time I needed to take care of myself," 44-year-old Kat wrote to me, "I realized fully that it was my responsibility to make it happen. Easier said than done," she concedes. But she does do it.

So do so many other women who have contacted me, all realizing that life is not going to get any less hectic and thus deciding that their health and well-being are priorities that need to take precedence over less pressing matters. Many make it happen by going to sleep a little earlier than most, which allows them to wake up earlier and fit "themselves" in then. Writes Sally, "my secret for staying strong is making time for myself. I am an attorney at a large law firm where the focus is on billable hours, making the environment very competitive and stressful. For both physical and emotional strength, I go to the gym at 5:30 every morning no matter how hard it may be to get out of bed. The hour or two I am at the gym is 'my time,' when everything else in my life takes a back seat—no meetings, no conference calls, no interruptions."

I wedge in time for myself by trying several days a week to walk the 23 minutes from the commuter train to my office and then back again at the end of the day (as long as it isn't 3 degrees outside). And I do at least one of my strength-training sessions on weekends, when the days are a bit less hectic.

Lack of time is the single most widely cited reason for why people don't participate in a regular physical activity program. But if you don't have time to take care of your body (which also includes time for shopping and preparing healthful meals), how can you possibly have time for anything else?

April

APRIL 1–7

I work in an industry that frequently requires long hours, but at least once a week I force myself to leave by 6 P.M., and I've set a rule for myself. If I leave the office by 6, I go to the gym. Frequently, I make it at least twice a week. And once there, I stay long enough to work off the day's or week's tension. I used to kill myself to get to the gym every day and was angry when I did not make it. I find that following my new rule is easy, and the results are still great.—CAROLINE

PERSONAL NOTES

APRIL 1, DAY OF THE WEEK S M T W TH F S

MOOD	VIGOR	SLEEP
	Excellent	
☐	☐	☐
☐	☐	☐
☐	☐	☐
	Poor	

APRIL 2, DAY OF THE WEEK S M T W TH F S

MOOD	VIGOR	SLEEP
	Excellent	
☐	☐	☐
☐	☐	☐
☐	☐	☐
	Poor	

APRIL 3, DAY OF THE WEEK S M T W TH F S

MOOD	VIGOR	SLEEP
	Excellent	
☐	☐	☐
☐	☐	☐
☐	☐	☐
	Poor	

For crispy chicken without the fatty skin, coat skinned chicken legs and wings in plain, nonfat yogurt, roll them in breadcrumbs, and bake in the oven. You'll get a delicious entrée—and some extra calcium with your dinner.

APRIL 4, DAY OF THE WEEK S M T W TH F S

MOOD	VIGOR	SLEEP
Excellent		
☐	☐	☐
☐	☐	☐
☐	☐	☐
Poor		

APRIL 5, DAY OF THE WEEK S M T W TH F S

MOOD	VIGOR	SLEEP
Excellent		
☐	☐	☐
☐	☐	☐
☐	☐	☐
Poor		

APRIL 6, DAY OF THE WEEK S M T W TH F S

MOOD	VIGOR	SLEEP
Excellent		
☐	☐	☐
☐	☐	☐
☐	☐	☐
Poor		

APRIL 7, DAY OF THE WEEK S M T W TH F S

MOOD	VIGOR	SLEEP
Excellent		
☐	☐	☐
☐	☐	☐
☐	☐	☐
Poor		

APRIL 1–7
NUTRITION LOG

GOALS (# SERVINGS)	WHOLE GRAINS	FRUITS	VEGETABLES	PROTEIN	DAIRY	EXTRAS
	3+	2+	3+	2–4	2–3	VARIABLE
APRIL 1	☐	☐	☐	☐	☐	☐
NOTES:						
APRIL 2	☐	☐	☐	☐	☐	☐
NOTES:						
APRIL 3	☐	☐	☐	☐	☐	☐
NOTES:						
APRIL 4	☐	☐	☐	☐	☐	☐
NOTES:						
APRIL 5	☐	☐	☐	☐	☐	☐
NOTES:						
APRIL 6	☐	☐	☐	☐	☐	☐
NOTES:						
APRIL 7	☐	☐	☐	☐	☐	☐
NOTES:						

CALCIUM + VITAMIN D ☐ VITAMIN E ☐ MULTIVITAMIN/MINERAL ☐

PLENTY OF FLUIDS ☐ OTHER SUPPLEMENTS _____

OVERALL COMMENTS

PHYSICAL ACTIVITY

planned, sport, leisure, errands, play
Goal: 30 to 60 minutes most days of the week

DAY	ACTIVITY	TIME

STRENGTH TRAINING

Goal: 2 to 3 times per week

EXERCISE 2 SETS/8 TO 10 REPS	DAY: POUNDS OR ✓	DAY: POUNDS OR ✓	DAY: POUNDS OR ✓

NUMBER OF STEPS

APRIL 1	APRIL 2	APRIL 3	APRIL 4	APRIL 5	APRIL 6	APRIL 7

APRIL 8–14

For those weaknesses that I want to improve upon, I have committed myself to working hard on them. For those weaknesses that I have decided are not priorities in my life, I have learned to let go of them and make no apologies for it. For example, I acknowledge that I am not as analytical or creative as some of my coworkers, but I focus on my personal strengths, which are organization and planning. I also know that I will never be a perfect size 8, but I can be fit and healthy and proud of my physical accomplishments, such as running a marathon or walking 60 miles for charity. The key to being a strong woman is to accept and respect yourself for who you are, continuously evaluate your priorities, set realistic goals, and work hard to achieve then.—SHARI

PERSONAL NOTES

APRIL 8, DAY OF THE WEEK   S   M   T   W   TH   F   S

MOOD	VIGOR	SLEEP
	Excellent	
☐	☐	☐
☐	☐	☐
☐	☐	☐
	Poor	

APRIL 9, DAY OF THE WEEK   S   M   T   W   TH   F   S

MOOD	VIGOR	SLEEP
	Excellent	
☐	☐	☐
☐	☐	☐
☐	☐	☐
	Poor	

APRIL 10, DAY OF THE WEEK   S   M   T   W   TH   F   S

MOOD	VIGOR	SLEEP
	Excellent	
☐	☐	☐
☐	☐	☐
☐	☐	☐
	Poor	

Keep packets of hot chocolate at the office to satisfy your sweet tooth. You'll save calories *and* money. A candy bar has about 250 calories and costs about 75 cents. A packet of hot chocolate has about 120 calories and costs roughly 20 cents.

APRIL 11, DAY OF THE WEEK   S   M   T   W   TH   F   S

MOOD	VIGOR	SLEEP
Excellent		
☐	☐	☐
☐	☐	☐
☐	☐	☐
Poor		

APRIL 12, DAY OF THE WEEK   S   M   T   W   TH   F   S

MOOD	VIGOR	SLEEP
Excellent		
☐	☐	☐
☐	☐	☐
☐	☐	☐
Poor		

APRIL 13, DAY OF THE WEEK   S   M   T   W   TH   F   S

MOOD	VIGOR	SLEEP
Excellent		
☐	☐	☐
☐	☐	☐
☐	☐	☐
Poor		

APRIL 14, DAY OF THE WEEK   S   M   T   W   TH   F   S

MOOD	VIGOR	SLEEP
Excellent		
☐	☐	☐
☐	☐	☐
☐	☐	☐
Poor		

APRIL 8–14
NUTRITION LOG

GOALS (# SERVINGS)	WHOLE GRAINS 3+	FRUITS 2+	VEGETABLES 3+	PROTEIN 2–4	DAIRY 2–3	EXTRAS VARIABLE
APRIL 8 NOTES:	☐	☐	☐	☐	☐	☐
APRIL 9 NOTES:	☐	☐	☐	☐	☐	☐
APRIL 10 NOTES:	☐	☐	☐	☐	☐	☐
APRIL 11 NOTES:	☐	☐	☐	☐	☐	☐
APRIL 12 NOTES:	☐	☐	☐	☐	☐	☐
APRIL 13 NOTES:	☐	☐	☐	☐	☐	☐
APRIL 14 NOTES:	☐	☐	☐	☐	☐	☐

CALCIUM + VITAMIN D ☐ **VITAMIN E** ☐ **MULTIVITAMIN/MINERAL** ☐

PLENTY OF FLUIDS ☐ **OTHER SUPPLEMENTS** _____

OVERALL COMMENTS

PHYSICAL ACTIVITY

planned, sport, leisure, errands, play
Goal: 30 to 60 minutes most days of the week

DAY	ACTIVITY	TIME

STRENGTH TRAINING

Goal: 2 to 3 times per week

EXERCISE 2 SETS/8 TO 10 REPS	DAY: POUNDS OR ✓	DAY: POUNDS OR ✓	DAY: POUNDS OR ✓

NUMBER OF STEPS

APRIL 8	APRIL 9	APRIL 10	APRIL 11	APRIL 12	APRIL 13	APRIL 14

APRIL 15–21

Last year at this time, I was cycling more than 30 miles a week, in addition to strength training three or four days weekly as well as daily stretching or yoga. I was in phenomenal condition. This year, I've endured an unreasonably busy work schedule, my father's death, moving to another state, and surgery for an ovarian cyst. I fit in workouts when I can. I'm not in the shape I was in last year and I have fewer plates on my barbell, but I'm okay with that. I've learned that some years are great, and some are just okay. My biceps may not be as defined as they were, but my inner strength is as developed as ever.—KIMBERLY

PERSONAL NOTES

APRIL 15, DAY OF THE WEEK S M T W TH F S

MOOD	VIGOR	SLEEP
Excellent		
☐	☐	☐
☐	☐	☐
☐	☐	☐
Poor		

APRIL 16, DAY OF THE WEEK S M T W TH F S

MOOD	VIGOR	SLEEP
Excellent		
☐	☐	☐
☐	☐	☐
☐	☐	☐
Poor		

APRIL 17, DAY OF THE WEEK S M T W TH F S

MOOD	VIGOR	SLEEP
Excellent		
☐	☐	☐
☐	☐	☐
☐	☐	☐
Poor		

If purchasing pre-made garden salads or already-cut fruit salads will make you more likely to eat them than if you have to cut up produce yourself, buy them even though they cost more. If you're worth the extra money for a pint of super-premium ice cream, you're certainly worth the extra money for something that will help improve your health.

APRIL 18, DAY OF THE WEEK   S   M   T   W   TH   F   S

	MOOD	VIGOR	SLEEP
	Excellent		
	☐	☐	☐
	☐	☐	☐
	☐	☐	☐
	Poor		

APRIL 19, DAY OF THE WEEK   S   M   T   W   TH   F   S

	MOOD	VIGOR	SLEEP
	Excellent		
	☐	☐	☐
	☐	☐	☐
	☐	☐	☐
	Poor		

APRIL 20, DAY OF THE WEEK   S   M   T   W   TH   F   S

	MOOD	VIGOR	SLEEP
	Excellent		
	☐	☐	☐
	☐	☐	☐
	☐	☐	☐
	Poor		

APRIL 21, DAY OF THE WEEK   S   M   T   W   TH   F   S

	MOOD	VIGOR	SLEEP
	Excellent		
	☐	☐	☐
	☐	☐	☐
	☐	☐	☐
	Poor		

APRIL 15–21
NUTRITION LOG

GOALS (# SERVINGS)	WHOLE GRAINS 3+	FRUITS 2+	VEGETABLES 3+	PROTEIN 2–4	DAIRY 2–3	EXTRAS VARIABLE
APRIL 15 NOTES:	☐	☐	☐	☐	☐	☐
APRIL 16 NOTES:	☐	☐	☐	☐	☐	☐
APRIL 17 NOTES:	☐	☐	☐	☐	☐	☐
APRIL 18 NOTES:	☐	☐	☐	☐	☐	☐
APRIL 19 NOTES:	☐	☐	☐	☐	☐	☐
APRIL 20 NOTES:	☐	☐	☐	☐	☐	☐
APRIL 21 NOTES:	☐	☐	☐	☐	☐	☐

CALCIUM + VITAMIN D ☐   VITAMIN E ☐   MULTIVITAMIN/MINERAL ☐

PLENTY OF FLUIDS ☐   OTHER SUPPLEMENTS _____

OVERALL COMMENTS

PHYSICAL ACTIVITY

planned, sport, leisure, errands, play
Goal: 30 to 60 minutes most days of the week

DAY	ACTIVITY	TIME

STRENGTH TRAINING

Goal: 2 to 3 times per week

EXERCISE 2 SETS/8 TO 10 REPS	DAY: POUNDS OR ✓	DAY: POUNDS OR ✓	DAY: POUNDS OR ✓

NUMBER OF STEPS

APRIL 15	APRIL 16	APRIL 17	APRIL 18	APRIL 19	APRIL 20	APRIL 21

APRIL 22–28

I grew up in a healthy, active family in Vermont. We grew an organic vegetable garden every summer, cross-country ski raced, and took ballet classes. It was a different kind of life. During the morning trek to school, I had to swing across a stream on a rope and scramble up an embankment. Then, as a teenager, I fell from a tree and became paralyzed from the waist down. To deal with the daily physical and emotional challenges of life in a wheelchair, I rely on the strength of my upbringing. I handcycle, put on my knobbies for a roll in the woods, stretch often, play guitar, and grow an organic garden. —ALICIA

PERSONAL NOTES

APRIL 22, DAY OF THE WEEK S M T W TH F S

MOOD	VIGOR	SLEEP
Excellent		
☐	☐	☐
☐	☐	☐
☐	☐	☐
Poor		

APRIL 23, DAY OF THE WEEK S M T W TH F S

MOOD	VIGOR	SLEEP
Excellent		
☐	☐	☐
☐	☐	☐
☐	☐	☐
Poor		

APRIL 24, DAY OF THE WEEK S M T W TH F S

MOOD	VIGOR	SLEEP
Excellent		
☐	☐	☐
☐	☐	☐
☐	☐	☐
Poor		

You don't need to eat red meat to have a healthful diet, but excluding red meat does not automatically make a diet healthful. In fact, red meat is high in iron and zinc, two nutrients that women, particularly during their childbearing years, don't get enough of. The trick is to keep portions smallish—3 ounces or so per serving (use the deck of cards comparison)—and alternate between red meat meals and other protein sources, including poultry, fish, beans, and tofu. Skewering a few pieces of meat onto kabobs with peppers, mushrooms, and other vegetables and then grilling them is a great way to keep portions small.

APRIL 25, DAY OF THE WEEK   S   M   T   W   TH   F   S

MOOD	VIGOR	SLEEP
	Excellent	
☐	☐	☐
☐	☐	☐
☐	☐	☐
	Poor	

APRIL 26, DAY OF THE WEEK   S   M   T   W   TH   F   S

MOOD	VIGOR	SLEEP
	Excellent	
☐	☐	☐
☐	☐	☐
☐	☐	☐
	Poor	

APRIL 27, DAY OF THE WEEK   S   M   T   W   TH   F   S

MOOD	VIGOR	SLEEP
	Excellent	
☐	☐	☐
☐	☐	☐
☐	☐	☐
	Poor	

APRIL 28, DAY OF THE WEEK   S   M   T   W   TH   F   S

MOOD	VIGOR	SLEEP
	Excellent	
☐	☐	☐
☐	☐	☐
☐	☐	☐
	Poor	

APRIL 22–28

NUTRITION LOG

GOALS (# SERVINGS)	WHOLE GRAINS 3+	FRUITS 2+	VEGETABLES 3+	PROTEIN 2–4	DAIRY 2–3	EXTRAS VARIABLE
APRIL 22 **NOTES:**	☐	☐	☐	☐	☐	☐
APRIL 23 **NOTES:**	☐	☐	☐	☐	☐	☐
APRIL 24 **NOTES:**	☐	☐	☐	☐	☐	☐
APRIL 25 **NOTES:**	☐	☐	☐	☐	☐	☐
APRIL 26 **NOTES:**	☐	☐	☐	☐	☐	☐
APRIL 27 **NOTES:**	☐	☐	☐	☐	☐	☐
APRIL 28 **NOTES:**	☐	☐	☐	☐	☐	☐

CALCIUM + VITAMIN D ☐ **VITAMIN E** ☐ **MULTIVITAMIN/MINERAL** ☐

PLENTY OF FLUIDS ☐ **OTHER SUPPLEMENTS** _____

OVERALL COMMENTS

PHYSICAL ACTIVITY

planned, sport, leisure, errands, play
Goal: 30 to 60 minutes most days of the week

DAY	ACTIVITY	TIME

STRENGTH TRAINING

Goal: 2 to 3 times per week

EXERCISE 2 SETS/8 TO 10 REPS	DAY: POUNDS OR ✓	DAY: POUNDS OR ✓	DAY: POUNDS OR ✓

NUMBER OF STEPS

APRIL 22   APRIL 23   APRIL 24   APRIL 25   APRIL 26   APRIL 27   APRIL 28

APRIL 29–30

PERSONAL NOTES

APRIL 29, DAY OF THE WEEK   S   M   T   W   TH   F   S

	MOOD	VIGOR	SLEEP
Excellent			
	☐	☐	☐
	☐	☐	☐
	☐	☐	☐
Poor			

APRIL 30, DAY OF THE WEEK   S   M   T   W   TH   F   S

	MOOD	VIGOR	SLEEP
Excellent			
	☐	☐	☐
	☐	☐	☐
	☐	☐	☐
Poor			

NUTRITION LOG

	WHOLE GRAINS	FRUITS	VEGETABLES	PROTEIN	DAIRY	EXTRAS
GOALS (# SERVINGS)	3+	2+	3+	2–4	2–3	VARIABLE
APRIL 29	☐	☐	☐	☐	☐	☐
NOTES:						
APRIL 30	☐	☐	☐	☐	☐	☐
NOTES:						

CALCIUM + VITAMIN D ☐   VITAMIN E ☐   MULTIVITAMIN/MINERAL ☐

PLENTY OF FLUIDS ☐   OTHER SUPPLEMENTS _____

OVERALL COMMENTS

PHYSICAL ACTIVITY

planned, sport, leisure, errands, play
Goal: 30 to 60 minutes most days of the week

DAY	ACTIVITY	TIME

STRENGTH TRAINING

Goal: 2 to 3 times per week

EXERCISE 2 SETS/8 TO 10 REPS	DAY: POUNDS OR ✓	DAY: POUNDS OR ✓	DAY: POUNDS OR ✓

NUMBER OF STEPS

APRIL 29   APRIL 30

_____   _____

APRIL REVIEW

BRIGHT SPOTS:

GREATEST CHALLENGES:

PATTERNS OBSERVED:

IDENTIFY BARRIERS TO CHANGE AND HOW I AM GOING TO OVERCOME THEM:

  PERSONAL

  PROFESSIONAL

PERSONAL CARE ATTENTION (flossing teeth, skin care, cutting/coloring hair, etc.):

WELLNESS CHECK (Did I have any sick days?):

BODY WEIGHT: MONTHLY CYCLE DATES (if applicable):

DOCTOR/DENTIST APPOINTMENTS:

MEDICATIONS TAKEN:

It's Not All Or Nothing

"When I don't have time for a 5-mile run," a woman named Chris said to me, "I often can find time for a 2-mile run. Being willing to do what you can, even when it is not what you want, is what it's all about."

Chris doesn't know how right she is. When it comes to exercise, the biggest gains in fitness come from doing something instead of nothing. Sure, the gains become even greater if you push yourself to do more. But there's a much more dramatic change in endurance and strength when you go from being sedentary to moderately active than from moderately active to very active. This finding has been seen over and over again in numerous scientific studies. That's why you absolutely should not make the mistake of foregoing exercise—on a particular day or in general—because you feel it wouldn't be enough to make a difference. Whatever you accomplish, even if it's less than usual or less than you would like, is much, much better for you than doing nothing at all.

It's the same with your eating strategy. If you can't follow through on all your ideas for eating a healthful diet, it's better to follow at least some of your plans rather than succumb to the false notion that eating well is an all-or-nothing proposition.

That's especially important to keep in mind at those times that you lapse in your exercise or nutrition program (and everyone does lapse sometimes). Many people, if they eat something they're not "supposed" to or engage in less physical activity than they planned, tell themselves they've "blown it" and completely give up their efforts. Giving up is the worst thing you can do—and one of the silliest, to boot. A single lapse, or even a few lapses, can't undo all the hard work that preceded it. Only mistakenly labeling a lapse a failure and then abandoning your program can do that.

May

MAY 1–7

I've begun to walk in the mornings with a woman who has Alzheimer's. She is 84 and absolutely gorgeous. As we start down the road, I like to ask her about her life, although when we begin, she often can't remember who her husband was or what he did for a living. A block or two later, she'll start to recall the way her mother looked the day they moved to America from Sweden. And just before we pass a statue in the park, she'll suddenly start to ramble on about her husband, only now she'll remember most everything about him and why it is she married him. We walk to a coffee shop three blocks further and order pecan rolls and coffee and laugh with the older, regular couples who stroll in. I can see a lifetime of courage and resilience in her eyes, and it puts life into perspective to sit there together. We give strength to each other, and at the end of our morning coffee, I feel young and strong and grateful for the day. Then I give her my hand, and we step back out into the world.—KATHERINE

PERSONAL NOTES

MAY 1, DAY OF THE WEEK   S   M   T   W   TH   F   S

MOOD	VIGOR	SLEEP
Excellent		
☐	☐	☐
☐	☐	☐
☐	☐	☐
Poor		

MAY 2, DAY OF THE WEEK   S   M   T   W   TH   F   S

MOOD	VIGOR	SLEEP
Excellent		
☐	☐	☐
☐	☐	☐
☐	☐	☐
Poor		

MAY 3, DAY OF THE WEEK   S   M   T   W   TH   F   S

MOOD	VIGOR	SLEEP
Excellent		
☐	☐	☐
☐	☐	☐
☐	☐	☐
Poor		

One way not to overeat is to get enough sleep! Preliminary research suggests that fatigue can lead to overeating. One theory is that when people are tired, they may eat to keep their bodies occupied and thereby avoid nodding off.

MAY 4, DAY OF THE WEEK S   M   T   W   TH   F   S

	MOOD	VIGOR	SLEEP
		Excellent	
	☐	☐	☐
	☐	☐	☐
	☐	☐	☐
		Poor	

MAY 5, DAY OF THE WEEK S   M   T   W   TH   F   S

	MOOD	VIGOR	SLEEP
		Excellent	
	☐	☐	☐
	☐	☐	☐
	☐	☐	☐
		Poor	

MAY 6, DAY OF THE WEEK S   M   T   W   TH   F   S

	MOOD	VIGOR	SLEEP
		Excellent	
	☐	☐	☐
	☐	☐	☐
	☐	☐	☐
		Poor	

MAY 7, DAY OF THE WEEK S   M   T   W   TH   F   S

	MOOD	VIGOR	SLEEP
		Excellent	
	☐	☐	☐
	☐	☐	☐
	☐	☐	☐
		Poor	

MAY 1–7
NUTRITION LOG

GOALS (# SERVINGS)	WHOLE GRAINS 3+	FRUITS 2+	VEGETABLES 3+	PROTEIN 2–4	DAIRY 2–3	EXTRAS VARIABLE
MAY 1 NOTES:	☐	☐	☐	☐	☐	☐
MAY 2 NOTES:	☐	☐	☐	☐	☐	☐
MAY 3 NOTES:	☐	☐	☐	☐	☐	☐
MAY 4 NOTES:	☐	☐	☐	☐	☐	☐
MAY 5 NOTES:	☐	☐	☐	☐	☐	☐
MAY 6 NOTES:	☐	☐	☐	☐	☐	☐
MAY 7 NOTES:	☐	☐	☐	☐	☐	☐

CALCIUM + VITAMIN D ☐　VITAMIN E ☐　MULTIVITAMIN/MINERAL ☐

PLENTY OF FLUIDS ☐　OTHER SUPPLEMENTS _____

OVERALL COMMENTS

PHYSICAL ACTIVITY

planned, sport, leisure, errands, play
Goal: 30 to 60 minutes most days of the week

DAY	ACTIVITY	TIME

STRENGTH TRAINING

Goal: 2 to 3 times per week

EXERCISE 2 SETS/8 TO 10 REPS	DAY: POUNDS OR ✓	DAY: POUNDS OR ✓	DAY: POUNDS OR ✓

NUMBER OF STEPS

MAY 1	MAY 2	MAY 3	MAY 4	MAY 5	MAY 6	MAY 7

May 8–14

*I am a process engineer at an aluminum shelter. My work is demanding, both physically and mentally. The job is hot and sweaty (I look like a wreck 10 hours a day), and I am constantly being pulled in several directions at once to get several things done. How do I stay strong physically and mentally? On the days I feel stressed, I take time to talk to our operators on the floor about matters unrelated to work (how their children are doing, what special things they have done lately). By reaching out to others in a nonwork-related manner, I build relationships and end up making someone smile before the day is over. This satisfaction is enough to keep me going.—*Valerie

Personal Notes

MAY 8, DAY OF THE WEEK   S   M   T   W   TH   F   S

MOOD	VIGOR	SLEEP
Excellent		
☐	☐	☐
☐	☐	☐
☐	☐	☐
Poor		

MAY 9, DAY OF THE WEEK   S   M   T   W   TH   F   S

MOOD	VIGOR	SLEEP
Excellent		
☐	☐	☐
☐	☐	☐
☐	☐	☐
Poor		

MAY 10, DAY OF THE WEEK   S   M   T   W   TH   F   S

MOOD	VIGOR	SLEEP
Excellent		
☐	☐	☐
☐	☐	☐
☐	☐	☐
Poor		

A half cup of cooked collard greens contains only 25 calories but provides 60 percent of the Daily Value for vitamin A (in the form of beta-carotene), 30 percent for vitamin C, and 20 percent for folate, not to mention some fiber. But these greens are "assertive" and can be bitter. To make fresh greens milder, drop them into a large pot of boiling water for about 10 minutes; press out excess moisture and chill under cold, running water; sauté some chopped onion and minced garlic in a little olive oil; then add collards and heat through. Season with lemon juice, and sprinkle with a few toasted almonds.

MAY 11, DAY OF THE WEEK   S   M   T   W   TH   F   S

MOOD	VIGOR	SLEEP
Excellent		
☐	☐	☐
☐	☐	☐
☐	☐	☐
Poor		

MAY 12, DAY OF THE WEEK   S   M   T   W   TH   F   S

MOOD	VIGOR	SLEEP
Excellent		
☐	☐	☐
☐	☐	☐
☐	☐	☐
Poor		

MAY 13, DAY OF THE WEEK   S   M   T   W   TH   F   S

MOOD	VIGOR	SLEEP
Excellent		
☐	☐	☐
☐	☐	☐
☐	☐	☐
Poor		

MAY 14, DAY OF THE WEEK   S   M   T   W   TH   F   S

MOOD	VIGOR	SLEEP
Excellent		
☐	☐	☐
☐	☐	☐
☐	☐	☐
Poor		

MAY 8–14
NUTRITION LOG

GOALS (# SERVINGS)	WHOLE GRAINS 3+	FRUITS 2+	VEGETABLES 3+	PROTEIN 2–4	DAIRY 2–3	EXTRAS VARIABLE
MAY 8 NOTES:	☐	☐	☐	☐	☐	☐
MAY 9 NOTES:	☐	☐	☐	☐	☐	☐
MAY 10 NOTES:	☐	☐	☐	☐	☐	☐
MAY 11 NOTES:	☐	☐	☐	☐	☐	☐
MAY 12 NOTES:	☐	☐	☐	☐	☐	☐
MAY 13 NOTES:	☐	☐	☐	☐	☐	☐
MAY 14 NOTES:	☐	☐	☐	☐	☐	☐

CALCIUM + VITAMIN D ☐ **VITAMIN E** ☐ **MULTIVITAMIN/MINERAL** ☐

PLENTY OF FLUIDS ☐ **OTHER SUPPLEMENTS** _____

OVERALL COMMENTS

PHYSICAL ACTIVITY

planned, sport, leisure, errands, play
Goal: 30 to 60 minutes most days of the week

DAY	ACTIVITY	TIME

STRENGTH TRAINING

Goal: 2 to 3 times per week

EXERCISE 2 SETS/8 TO 10 REPS	DAY: POUNDS OR ✓	DAY: POUNDS OR ✓	DAY: POUNDS OR ✓

NUMBER OF STEPS

MAY 8	MAY 9	MAY 10	MAY 11	MAY 12	MAY 13	MAY 14

MAY 15–21

Two years ago I fell on a patch of ice and broke my ankle in three places. After four months in a wheelchair, I struggled with residual pain in my ankle and back, making walking difficult. It wasn't long before the lack of exercise added a hundred extra pounds to my frame. Knowing obesity, diabetes, and high blood pressure are common in my family, I decided it was time to take action. I joined a health club with a friend who also wanted to lose weight. Together we have been taking daily walks, gradually increasing the distance I can tolerate. We swim and exercise together at the health club and shop together for healthy food. Our goal is not merely weight loss, but to improve our overall health through better nutrition and exercise. With the support of each other, we are finding we can do together what neither of us could do alone. Each day I find myself becoming a little stronger.—LISA

PERSONAL NOTES

MAY 15, DAY OF THE WEEK   S   M   T   W   TH   F   S

MOOD	VIGOR	SLEEP
Excellent		
☐	☐	☐
☐	☐	☐
☐	☐	☐
Poor		

MAY 16, DAY OF THE WEEK   S   M   T   W   TH   F   S

MOOD	VIGOR	SLEEP
Excellent		
☐	☐	☐
☐	☐	☐
☐	☐	☐
Poor		

MAY 17, DAY OF THE WEEK   S   M   T   W   TH   F   S

MOOD	VIGOR	SLEEP
Excellent		
☐	☐	☐
☐	☐	☐
☐	☐	☐
Poor		

Over 60? Predict your risk of suffering a serious fall by balancing on one leg (while bending the other at the knee). If you're not able to stand on one leg for at least five seconds, you're at more than double the risk of hurting yourself in a fall than someone your age who can, says a study from the University of New Mexico. The good news: Targeted exercises such as one-legged stands, tandem walking (walking in a straight line with one foot in front of the other), and various yoga poses can improve balance and coordination and substantially ratchet down the risk.

MAY 18, DAY OF THE WEEK   S   M   T   W   TH   F   S

MOOD	VIGOR	SLEEP
Excellent		
☐	☐	☐
☐	☐	☐
☐	☐	☐
Poor		

MAY 19, DAY OF THE WEEK   S   M   T   W   TH   F   S

MOOD	VIGOR	SLEEP
Excellent		
☐	☐	☐
☐	☐	☐
☐	☐	☐
Poor		

MAY 20, DAY OF THE WEEK   S   M   T   W   TH   F   S

MOOD	VIGOR	SLEEP
Excellent		
☐	☐	☐
☐	☐	☐
☐	☐	☐
Poor		

MAY 21, DAY OF THE WEEK   S   M   T   W   TH   F   S

MOOD	VIGOR	SLEEP
Excellent		
☐	☐	☐
☐	☐	☐
☐	☐	☐
Poor		

MAY 15–21
NUTRITION LOG

GOALS (# SERVINGS)	WHOLE GRAINS 3+	FRUITS 2+	VEGETABLES 3+	PROTEIN 2–4	DAIRY 2–3	EXTRAS VARIABLE
MAY 15	☐	☐	☐	☐	☐	☐
NOTES:						
MAY 16	☐	☐	☐	☐	☐	☐
NOTES:						
MAY 17	☐	☐	☐	☐	☐	☐
NOTES:						
MAY 18	☐	☐	☐	☐	☐	☐
NOTES:						
MAY 19	☐	☐	☐	☐	☐	☐
NOTES:						
MAY 20	☐	☐	☐	☐	☐	☐
NOTES:						
MAY 21	☐	☐	☐	☐	☐	☐
NOTES:						

CALCIUM + VITAMIN D ☐ **VITAMIN E** ☐ **MULTIVITAMIN/MINERAL** ☐

PLENTY OF FLUIDS ☐ **OTHER SUPPLEMENTS** _____

OVERALL COMMENTS

PHYSICAL ACTIVITY

planned, sport, leisure, errands, play
Goal: 30 to 60 minutes most days of the week

DAY	ACTIVITY	TIME

STRENGTH TRAINING

Goal: 2 to 3 times per week

EXERCISE 2 SETS/8 TO 10 REPS	DAY: POUNDS OR ✓	DAY: POUNDS OR ✓	DAY: POUNDS OR ✓

NUMBER OF STEPS

MAY 15	MAY 16	MAY 17	MAY 18	MAY 19	MAY 20	MAY 21

MAY 22–28

*During this past year, a supportive companion, a strong sense of end goal, and confidence in my own will and abilities helped me come through some challenging goals triumphantly. It was a year ago that my husband and I started trying to conceive, but I had been diagnosed with polycystic ovarian syndrome, making conception difficult. Through all the negative pregnancy tests and various medications, my husband reaffirmed his love and support for me. At the same time, I made the decision to make changes to my diet and also to exercise. I wanted a healthy body for me and (hopefully) my future baby. When I ate something not healthy or skipped a workout, I held myself accountable, but I didn't let it hold me back; the next day was a new day. A year later I'm thrilled to report that I'm exercising regularly, I've lost 10 pounds, and, most importantly, I became pregnant!—*ZEHAVA

PERSONAL NOTES

MAY 22, DAY OF THE WEEK S M T W TH F S

MOOD	VIGOR	SLEEP
Excellent		
☐	☐	☐
☐	☐	☐
☐	☐	☐
Poor		

MAY 23, DAY OF THE WEEK S M T W TH F S

MOOD	VIGOR	SLEEP
Excellent		
☐	☐	☐
☐	☐	☐
☐	☐	☐
Poor		

MAY 24, DAY OF THE WEEK S M T W TH F S

MOOD	VIGOR	SLEEP
Excellent		
☐	☐	☐
☐	☐	☐
☐	☐	☐
Poor		

Exercise is good for the brain! People who exercise regularly throughout their lives appear to maintain their memory function better than sedentary people. The thinking is that exercise helps pump oxygen to the brain, where it's needed to keep nerve cells functioning properly.

MAY 25, DAY OF THE WEEK   S   M   T   W   TH   F   S

MOOD	VIGOR	SLEEP
Excellent		
☐	☐	☐
☐	☐	☐
☐	☐	☐
Poor		

MAY 26, DAY OF THE WEEK   S   M   T   W   TH   F   S

MOOD	VIGOR	SLEEP
Excellent		
☐	☐	☐
☐	☐	☐
☐	☐	☐
Poor		

MAY 27, DAY OF THE WEEK   S   M   T   W   TH   F   S

MOOD	VIGOR	SLEEP
Excellent		
☐	☐	☐
☐	☐	☐
☐	☐	☐
Poor		

MAY 28, DAY OF THE WEEK   S   M   T   W   TH   F   S

MOOD	VIGOR	SLEEP
Excellent		
☐	☐	☐
☐	☐	☐
☐	☐	☐
Poor		

MAY 22–28
NUTRITION LOG

GOALS (# SERVINGS)	WHOLE GRAINS 3+	FRUITS 2+	VEGETABLES 3+	PROTEIN 2–4	DAIRY 2–3	EXTRAS VARIABLE
MAY 22 NOTES:	☐	☐	☐	☐	☐	☐
MAY 23 NOTES:	☐	☐	☐	☐	☐	☐
MAY 24 NOTES:	☐	☐	☐	☐	☐	☐
MAY 25 NOTES:	☐	☐	☐	☐	☐	☐
MAY 26 NOTES:	☐	☐	☐	☐	☐	☐
MAY 27 NOTES:	☐	☐	☐	☐	☐	☐
MAY 28 NOTES:	☐	☐	☐	☐	☐	☐

CALCIUM + VITAMIN D ☐ VITAMIN E ☐ MULTIVITAMIN/MINERAL ☐

PLENTY OF FLUIDS ☐ OTHER SUPPLEMENTS _____

OVERALL COMMENTS

PHYSICAL ACTIVITY

planned, sport, leisure, errands, play
Goal: 30 to 60 minutes most days of the week

DAY	ACTIVITY	TIME

STRENGTH TRAINING

Goal: 2 to 3 times per week

EXERCISE 2 SETS/8 TO 10 REPS	DAY: POUNDS OR ✓	DAY: POUNDS OR ✓	DAY: POUNDS OR ✓

NUMBER OF STEPS

MAY 22	MAY 23	MAY 24	MAY 25	MAY 26	MAY 27	MAY 28

MAY 29–31

PERSONAL NOTES

MAY 29, DAY OF THE WEEK S M T W TH F S

MOOD	VIGOR	SLEEP
Excellent		
☐	☐	☐
☐	☐	☐
☐	☐	☐
Poor		

MAY 30, DAY OF THE WEEK S M T W TH F S

MOOD	VIGOR	SLEEP
Excellent		
☐	☐	☐
☐	☐	☐
☐	☐	☐
Poor		

MAY 31, DAY OF THE WEEK S M T W TH F S

MOOD	VIGOR	SLEEP
Excellent		
☐	☐	☐
☐	☐	☐
☐	☐	☐
Poor		

MAY 29–31
NUTRITION LOG

	WHOLE GRAINS	FRUITS	VEGETABLES	PROTEIN	DAIRY	EXTRAS
GOALS (# SERVINGS)	3+	2+	3+	2–4	2–3	VARIABLE
MAY 29	☐	☐	☐	☐	☐	☐
NOTES:						
MAY 30	☐	☐	☐	☐	☐	☐
NOTES:						
MAY 31	☐	☐	☐	☐	☐	☐
NOTES:						

CALCIUM + VITAMIN D ☐   VITAMIN E ☐   MULTIVITAMIN/MINERAL ☐

PLENTY OF FLUIDS ☐   OTHER SUPPLEMENTS _____

OVERALL COMMENTS

PHYSICAL ACTIVITY

planned, sport, leisure, errands, play
Goal: 30 to 60 minutes most days of the week

DAY	ACTIVITY	TIME

STRENGTH TRAINING

Goal: 2 to 3 times per week

EXERCISE 2 SETS/8 TO 10 REPS	DAY: POUNDS OR ✓	DAY: POUNDS OR ✓	DAY: POUNDS OR ✓

NUMBER OF STEPS

MAY 29   MAY 30   MAY 31

_____   _____   _____

MAY REVIEW

BRIGHT SPOTS:
_____

GREATEST CHALLENGES:
_____
_____
_____

PATTERNS OBSERVED:
_____

IDENTIFY BARRIERS TO CHANGE AND HOW I AM GOING TO OVERCOME THEM:

    PERSONAL
_____
_____

    PROFESSIONAL
_____
_____

PERSONAL CARE ATTENTION (flossing teeth, skin care, cutting/coloring hair, etc.):
_____
_____

WELLNESS CHECK (Did I have any sick days?):
_____
_____

BODY WEIGHT: MONTHLY CYCLE DATES (if applicable):
_____

DOCTOR/DENTIST APPOINTMENTS:
_____
_____

MEDICATIONS TAKEN:
_____
_____
_____

On Intimacy

✦

"*My husband is my best friend. He makes me laugh. Whenever things go wrong, I know he is there to support me.*"

"*Every morning, as I'm getting ready for the hectic day ahead of me, I pray to the Lord to help me and all the people I love. Spending time with God helps me face everyday challenges and stresses.*"

"*We named our circle of five 'Spa Sisters' because we indulge in a weekly relaxation ritual of lap swimming, Jacuzzi soak, and sauna before our kundalini yoga class. This is a necessity for us working women to maintain our sanity during a busy and stressful week, not to mention a wonderful way to catch up on each other's lives.*"

As you can see, intimacy comes in all shapes and sizes. But however it comes, it's crucial. As 25-year-old Amy, a woman wise beyond her years, said to me, "a woman of strength builds relationships to keep her soul in shape."

I count myself very lucky on the intimacy front. I have a loving husband and three wonderful children. I'm also lucky enough to still have my parents and in-laws, along with a number of close friends. At bottom, it's close personal contact with people I love, intimacy, that keeps me going. Indeed, intimacy, love, caring for another human being—whatever you want to call it—has been linked to good health and longevity.

I urge all of you to find intimacy in your lives if you don't already have it. If you live alone, join a club, house of worship, or community center—anything that will put you in touch with people. If you feel lonely more often than not, reach out by inviting someone to dinner or suggesting another way to spend time together. It might be hard to do at first, and not all efforts will turn into friendships. But *some* will. And your mental *and* physical health will benefit from having made the connections.

June

JUNE 1-7

I stand at the pool's edge, stretching my freshly wakened limbs, black cap and goggles giving me a formidable, almost alien look. Anticipating the initial shock of the cool water on my warm body, I dip one foot in the crystal-clear liquid to test the temperature before diving into the deep end of the pool. In an Alice in Wonderland *moment, the real world is abruptly left behind, and I enter that wonderful, aquatic, womb-like world where everything is peaceful and surreal. One hundred laps later, I make my way to the ladder and slowly climb out of the pool. Like a miraculous salve for the unmerciful wounds that life inflicts, any stress, worry, or hurt has been magically washed away by the cool, clear other-world from which I reluctantly pull myself.*—SUSAN

PERSONAL NOTES

JUNE 1, DAY OF THE WEEK   S   M   T   W   TH   F   S

MOOD	VIGOR	SLEEP
	Excellent	
☐	☐	☐
☐	☐	☐
☐	☐	☐
	Poor	

JUNE 2, DAY OF THE WEEK   S   M   T   W   TH   F   S

MOOD	VIGOR	SLEEP
	Excellent	
☐	☐	☐
☐	☐	☐
☐	☐	☐
	Poor	

JUNE 3, DAY OF THE WEEK   S   M   T   W   TH   F   S

MOOD	VIGOR	SLEEP
	Excellent	
☐	☐	☐
☐	☐	☐
☐	☐	☐
	Poor	

An ounce of Asiago cheese has 120 calories but also 25 percent of the Daily Value for calcium. Try pairing a bit of the piquant cheese (which has a nutty, pleasantly salted flavor) with a couple of figs, some grapes, an apple, or a pear. It will make for a delicious, healthful dessert or hearty snack. Edam cheese, with a similar nutrition profile, goes well with peaches, apricots, and cherries.

JUNE 4, DAY OF THE WEEK   S   M   T   W   TH   F   S

MOOD	VIGOR	SLEEP
Excellent		
☐	☐	☐
☐	☐	☐
☐	☐	☐
Poor		

JUNE 5, DAY OF THE WEEK   S   M   T   W   TH   F   S

MOOD	VIGOR	SLEEP
Excellent		
☐	☐	☐
☐	☐	☐
☐	☐	☐
Poor		

JUNE 6, DAY OF THE WEEK   S   M   T   W   TH   F   S

MOOD	VIGOR	SLEEP
Excellent		
☐	☐	☐
☐	☐	☐
☐	☐	☐
Poor		

JUNE 7, DAY OF THE WEEK   S   M   T   W   TH   F   S

MOOD	VIGOR	SLEEP
Excellent		
☐	☐	☐
☐	☐	☐
☐	☐	☐
Poor		

JUNE 1–7

NUTRITION LOG

GOALS (# SERVINGS)	WHOLE GRAINS 3+	FRUITS 2+	VEGETABLES 3+	PROTEIN 2–4	DAIRY 2–3	EXTRAS VARIABLE
JUNE 1	☐	☐	☐	☐	☐	☐
NOTES:						
JUNE 2	☐	☐	☐	☐	☐	☐
NOTES:						
JUNE 3	☐	☐	☐	☐	☐	☐
NOTES:						
JUNE 4	☐	☐	☐	☐	☐	☐
NOTES:						
JUNE 5	☐	☐	☐	☐	☐	☐
NOTES:						
JUNE 6	☐	☐	☐	☐	☐	☐
NOTES:						
JUNE 7	☐	☐	☐	☐	☐	☐
NOTES:						

CALCIUM + VITAMIN D ☐   VITAMIN E ☐   MULTIVITAMIN/MINERAL ☐

PLENTY OF FLUIDS ☐   OTHER SUPPLEMENTS _____

OVERALL COMMENTS

PHYSICAL ACTIVITY

planned, sport, leisure, errands, play
Goal: 30 to 60 minutes most days of the week

DAY	ACTIVITY	TIME

STRENGTH TRAINING

Goal: 2 to 3 times per week

EXERCISE 2 SETS/8 TO 10 REPS	DAY: POUNDS OR ✓	DAY: POUNDS OR ✓	DAY: POUNDS OR ✓

NUMBER OF STEPS

JUNE 1	JUNE 2	JUNE 3	JUNE 4	JUNE 5	JUNE 6	JUNE 7

JUNE 8–14

My mother and her twin sister are 81 and going strong. Unfortunately, their bodies are not in as good shape as their constitutions. After watching my mother have to pull herself up stairs because she could not lift her legs high enough to step up without assistance, I vowed not to have lost my strength when I'm 80. So I walk five times a week, take a 1½-hour Pilates class each week, and lift weights. I also try to park away from my mall destination, do an extra lap when I'm there, and take the stairs whenever possible. When I have to take an elevator or escalator, I pull in my stomach and clench my glutes. In other words, the things I do are not remarkable. Nor are they difficult. I have a weight bar and ball at home but no expensive workout equipment.—MARILYN

PERSONAL NOTES

JUNE 8, DAY OF THE WEEK   S   M   T   W   TH   F   S

MOOD	VIGOR	SLEEP
Excellent		
☐	☐	☐
☐	☐	☐
☐	☐	☐
Poor		

JUNE 9, DAY OF THE WEEK   S   M   T   W   TH   F   S

MOOD	VIGOR	SLEEP
Excellent		
☐	☐	☐
☐	☐	☐
☐	☐	☐
Poor		

JUNE 10, DAY OF THE WEEK   S   M   T   W   TH   F   S

MOOD	VIGOR	SLEEP
Excellent		
☐	☐	☐
☐	☐	☐
☐	☐	☐
Poor		

Exercising your abdominals isn't just for trying to achieve a washboard stomach. Having strong abdominals is also linked to better bone density, which can help prevent fractures. And it improves balance by helping to maintain the stability of the body's trunk. Abdominal curls and pelvic tilts are both good abdominal exercises. Try them a few times a week along with back extension exercises to give the other side of your body's scaffolding a workout as well.

JUNE 11, DAY OF THE WEEK   S   M   T   W   TH   F   S

MOOD	VIGOR	SLEEP
Excellent		
□	□	□
□	□	□
□	□	□
Poor		

JUNE 12, DAY OF THE WEEK   S   M   T   W   TH   F   S

MOOD	VIGOR	SLEEP
Excellent		
□	□	□
□	□	□
□	□	□
Poor		

JUNE 13, DAY OF THE WEEK   S   M   T   W   TH   F   S

MOOD	VIGOR	SLEEP
Excellent		
□	□	□
□	□	□
□	□	□
Poor		

JUNE 14, DAY OF THE WEEK   S   M   T   W   TH   F   S

MOOD	VIGOR	SLEEP
Excellent		
□	□	□
□	□	□
□	□	□
Poor		

JUNE 8–14
NUTRITION LOG

GOALS (# SERVINGS)	WHOLE GRAINS 3+	FRUITS 2+	VEGETABLES 3+	PROTEIN 2–4	DAIRY 2–3	EXTRAS VARIABLE
JUNE 8	☐	☐	☐	☐	☐	☐
NOTES:						
JUNE 9	☐	☐	☐	☐	☐	☐
NOTES:						
JUNE 10	☐	☐	☐	☐	☐	☐
NOTES:						
JUNE 11	☐	☐	☐	☐	☐	☐
NOTES:						
JUNE 12	☐	☐	☐	☐	☐	☐
NOTES:						
JUNE 13	☐	☐	☐	☐	☐	☐
NOTES:						
JUNE 14	☐	☐	☐	☐	☐	☐
NOTES:						

CALCIUM + VITAMIN D ☐   VITAMIN E ☐   MULTIVITAMIN/MINERAL ☐

PLENTY OF FLUIDS ☐   OTHER SUPPLEMENTS _____

OVERALL COMMENTS

PHYSICAL ACTIVITY

planned, sport, leisure, errands, play
Goal: 30 to 60 minutes most days of the week

DAY	ACTIVITY	TIME

STRENGTH TRAINING

Goal: 2 to 3 times per week

EXERCISE 2 SETS/8 TO 10 REPS	DAY: POUNDS OR ✓	DAY: POUNDS OR ✓	DAY: POUNDS OR ✓

NUMBER OF STEPS

JUNE 8	JUNE 9	JUNE 10	JUNE 11	JUNE 12	JUNE 13	JUNE 14

JUNE 15-21

Although the 1960s was a time of social upheaval, petite and pretty was still the standard for girls, not strong and muscular. Growing up in suburban Connecticut, it didn't occur to me that I shouldn't run as fast or climb as many trees as my four brothers. There is a photograph of me as a teenager, standing next to my brother's girlfriend. I look like an Amazon, tanned and fit, compared to her. I did not receive positive feedback for that image, to put it mildly. Slender and petite is not my body type. I spent a lot of time fighting this mental image before allowing myself the permission to like my body. What a refreshing and liberating concept! It's much more fun to be the strongest person in my fitness class (and one of the oldest to boot). I like hearing older women respond with surprise and pleasure at the declaration of my middle-aged strength and really like being able to hold my own playing tennis against younger women. Getting older is much more fun than I thought it was going to be. Strong Women Rule!—THERESE

PERSONAL NOTES

JUNE 15, DAY OF THE WEEK   S   M   T   W   TH   F   S

MOOD	VIGOR	SLEEP
Excellent		
□	□	□
□	□	□
□	□	□
Poor		

JUNE 16, DAY OF THE WEEK   S   M   T   W   TH   F   S

MOOD	VIGOR	SLEEP
Excellent		
□	□	□
□	□	□
□	□	□
Poor		

JUNE 17, DAY OF THE WEEK   S   M   T   W   TH   F   S

MOOD	VIGOR	SLEEP
Excellent		
□	□	□
□	□	□
□	□	□
Poor		

Practicing tai chi reduces stress because of its slow, graceful movements. But it's even known to reduce the body's levels of cortisol, a fight-or-flight hormone involved in stress. You don't have to take a tai chi class to learn this gentle martial arts form. You can rent a tai chi video from the library.

JUNE 18, DAY OF THE WEEK   S   M   T   W   TH   F   S

MOOD	VIGOR	SLEEP
Excellent		
□	□	□
□	□	□
□	□	□
Poor		

JUNE 19, DAY OF THE WEEK   S   M   T   W   TH   F   S

MOOD	VIGOR	SLEEP
Excellent		
□	□	□
□	□	□
□	□	□
Poor		

JUNE 20, DAY OF THE WEEK   S   M   T   W   TH   F   S

MOOD	VIGOR	SLEEP
Excellent		
□	□	□
□	□	□
□	□	□
Poor		

JUNE 21, DAY OF THE WEEK   S   M   T   W   TH   F   S

MOOD	VIGOR	SLEEP
Excellent		
□	□	□
□	□	□
□	□	□
Poor		

JUNE 15–21
NUTRITION LOG

GOALS (# SERVINGS)	WHOLE GRAINS	FRUITS	VEGETABLES	PROTEIN	DAIRY	EXTRAS
	3+	2+	3+	2–4	2–3	VARIABLE
JUNE 15	☐	☐	☐	☐	☐	☐
NOTES:						
JUNE 16	☐	☐	☐	☐	☐	☐
NOTES:						
JUNE 17	☐	☐	☐	☐	☐	☐
NOTES:						
JUNE 18	☐	☐	☐	☐	☐	☐
NOTES:						
JUNE 19	☐	☐	☐	☐	☐	☐
NOTES:						
JUNE 20	☐	☐	☐	☐	☐	☐
NOTES:						
JUNE 21	☐	☐	☐	☐	☐	☐
NOTES:						

CALCIUM + VITAMIN D ☐ **VITAMIN E** ☐ **MULTIVITAMIN/MINERAL** ☐

PLENTY OF FLUIDS ☐ **OTHER SUPPLEMENTS** _____

OVERALL COMMENTS

PHYSICAL ACTIVITY

planned, sport, leisure, errands, play
Goal: 30 to 60 minutes most days of the week

DAY	ACTIVITY	TIME

STRENGTH TRAINING

Goal: 2 to 3 times per week

EXERCISE 2 SETS/8 TO 10 REPS	DAY: POUNDS OR ✓	DAY: POUNDS OR ✓	DAY: POUNDS OR ✓

NUMBER OF STEPS

JUNE 15	JUNE 16	JUNE 17	JUNE 18	JUNE 19	JUNE 20	JUNE 21

JUNE 22–28

Focus on a small part of the situation, upon which you can have an effect, and take positive action. After you have taken that first step, the entire situation may appear more manageable. You can begin by holding your pulse point and counting just a little bit slower than your heart is beating while you breathe deeply and slowly. Notice as your pulse adjusts itself to your counting. Imagine yourself in a safe and supportive environment—perhaps in a hammock between palm trees in the Caribbean, swinging slowly in the breeze. As you become calm, you can slowly emerge and approach the situation with a relaxed body and a clear mind. The more you practice, the easier it becomes. Try it now. "The sky is blue overhead. I am in my hammock . . ."—CAROLINE

PERSONAL NOTES

JUNE 22, DAY OF THE WEEK   S   M   T   W   TH   F   S

MOOD	VIGOR	SLEEP
Excellent		
☐	☐	☐
☐	☐	☐
☐	☐	☐
Poor		

JUNE 23, DAY OF THE WEEK   S   M   T   W   TH   F   S

MOOD	VIGOR	SLEEP
Excellent		
☐	☐	☐
☐	☐	☐
☐	☐	☐
Poor		

JUNE 24, DAY OF THE WEEK   S   M   T   W   TH   F   S

MOOD	VIGOR	SLEEP
Excellent		
☐	☐	☐
☐	☐	☐
☐	☐	☐
Poor		

Never eat in the car. You deserve to savor your meals and snacks in a relaxed atmosphere, not simply swallow them.

JUNE 25, DAY OF THE WEEK S M T W TH F S

MOOD	VIGOR	SLEEP
	Excellent	
☐	☐	☐
☐	☐	☐
☐	☐	☐
	Poor	

JUNE 26, DAY OF THE WEEK S M T W TH F S

MOOD	VIGOR	SLEEP
	Excellent	
☐	☐	☐
☐	☐	☐
☐	☐	☐
	Poor	

JUNE 27, DAY OF THE WEEK S M T W TH F S

MOOD	VIGOR	SLEEP
	Excellent	
☐	☐	☐
☐	☐	☐
☐	☐	☐
	Poor	

JUNE 28, DAY OF THE WEEK S M T W TH F S

MOOD	VIGOR	SLEEP
	Excellent	
☐	☐	☐
☐	☐	☐
☐	☐	☐
	Poor	

JUNE 22–28
NUTRITION LOG

GOALS (# SERVINGS)	WHOLE GRAINS 3+	FRUITS 2+	VEGETABLES 3+	PROTEIN 2–4	DAIRY 2–3	EXTRAS VARIABLE
JUNE 22	☐	☐	☐	☐	☐	☐
NOTES:						
JUNE 23	☐	☐	☐	☐	☐	☐
NOTES:						
JUNE 24	☐	☐	☐	☐	☐	☐
NOTES:						
JUNE 25	☐	☐	☐	☐	☐	☐
NOTES:						
JUNE 26	☐	☐	☐	☐	☐	☐
NOTES:						
JUNE 27	☐	☐	☐	☐	☐	☐
NOTES:						
JUNE 28	☐	☐	☐	☐	☐	☐
NOTES:						

CALCIUM + VITAMIN D ☐ VITAMIN E ☐ MULTIVITAMIN/MINERAL ☐

PLENTY OF FLUIDS ☐ OTHER SUPPLEMENTS _____

OVERALL COMMENTS

PHYSICAL ACTIVITY

planned, sport, leisure, errands, play
Goal: 30 to 60 minutes most days of the week

DAY	ACTIVITY	TIME

STRENGTH TRAINING

Goal: 2 to 3 times per week

EXERCISE 2 SETS/8 TO 10 REPS	DAY: POUNDS OR ✓	DAY: POUNDS OR ✓	DAY: POUNDS OR ✓

NUMBER OF STEPS

JUNE 22	JUNE 23	JUNE 24	JUNE 25	JUNE 26	JUNE 27	JUNE 28

JUNE 29–30

PERSONAL NOTES

JUNE 29, DAY OF THE WEEK   S   M   T   W   TH   F   S

	MOOD	VIGOR	SLEEP
Excellent			
	☐	☐	☐
	☐	☐	☐
	☐	☐	☐
Poor			

JUNE 30, DAY OF THE WEEK   S   M   T   W   TH   F   S

	MOOD	VIGOR	SLEEP
Excellent			
	☐	☐	☐
	☐	☐	☐
	☐	☐	☐
Poor			

NUTRITION LOG

	WHOLE GRAINS	FRUITS	VEGETABLES	PROTEIN	DAIRY	EXTRAS
GOALS (# SERVINGS)	3+	2+	3+	2–4	2–3	VARIABLE
JUNE 29	☐	☐	☐	☐	☐	☐
NOTES:						
JUNE 30	☐	☐	☐	☐	☐	☐
NOTES:						

CALCIUM + VITAMIN D ☐   VITAMIN E ☐   MULTIVITAMIN/MINERAL ☐

PLENTY OF FLUIDS ☐   OTHER SUPPLEMENTS _____

OVERALL COMMENTS

PHYSICAL ACTIVITY

planned, sport, leisure, errands, play
Goal: 30 to 60 minutes most days of the week

DAY	ACTIVITY	TIME

STRENGTH TRAINING

Goal: 2 to 3 times per week

EXERCISE 2 SETS/8 TO 10 REPS	DAY: POUNDS OR ✓	DAY: POUNDS OR ✓	DAY: POUNDS OR ✓

NUMBER OF STEPS

JUNE 29   JUNE 30

_____   _____

JUNE REVIEW

BRIGHT SPOTS:
_____

GREATEST CHALLENGES:
_____
_____

PATTERNS OBSERVED:
_____

IDENTIFY BARRIERS TO CHANGE AND HOW I AM GOING TO OVERCOME THEM:

    PERSONAL
_____
_____

    PROFESSIONAL
_____
_____

PERSONAL CARE ATTENTION (flossing teeth, skin care, cutting/coloring hair, etc.):
_____
_____

WELLNESS CHECK (Did I have any sick days?):
_____
_____

BODY WEIGHT: MONTHLY CYCLE DATES (if applicable):
_____

DOCTOR/DENTIST APPOINTMENTS:
_____
_____

MEDICATIONS TAKEN:
_____
_____

Visualize It

❧

Have you ever visualized yourself in a place you're not? Perhaps it was on a tropical island, or in a pair of size six pants, or at the finish line of a long race. Experts say that imagining yourself where you want to be can be a very motivating force for helping you to stay on track so you can get there.

Visualization is very big in competitive sports. In fact, there's even a book called *Imagery Training in Sports*, in which it's recommended that you call up the image of yourself succeeding over and over, involving all your senses, as preparation for reaching your goal. I have found that visualization works for reaching all kinds of goals. So have many of the women who have contacted me.

Comments Mona, "I keep my life strong by believing that I can shape it in the direction that I choose, by focusing on creative visualization." Another woman wrote to me that she keeps herself strong "emotionally and physically by taking time out to go for a walk in the morning before sunrise. The streets are quiet," she said, "and there is little traffic, which allows me to think over the day and visualize myself handling tough situations in a positive way." That is, she visualizes so she can cope with day-to-day snags as they arise. Similarly, Zoë wrote, "I visualize the answers to challenges and set a plan in motion, then do it."

Visualization can work on any number of levels, from imagining yourself refusing a second helping of dessert from an insistent hostess, to being a stronger person once you start strength training, to calmly refusing to give in to a boss who is making unfair requests of you. I find it works best if you can sit in a quiet place without interruption, take some deep breaths to relax, close your eyes, and "roll a tape" that shows you succeeding.

July

JULY 1–7

I was not enjoying my high-pressure sales job, so I switched my office to a cubicle and took a pay cut. The benefit is that I can leave work at 5 o'clock and not have to worry about anything in the evening except my workout. I am enjoying this way of life so much more because I am being true to myself. It is not easy to explain to friends and coworkers why I am stepping down the corporate ladder, but in my heart it feels right, and I trust that feeling despite any doubts others may have.—KRISTIN

PERSONAL NOTES

JULY 1, DAY OF THE WEEK   S   M   T   W   TH   F   S

MOOD	VIGOR	SLEEP
Excellent		
☐	☐	☐
☐	☐	☐
☐	☐	☐
Poor		

JULY 2, DAY OF THE WEEK   S   M   T   W   TH   F   S

MOOD	VIGOR	SLEEP
Excellent		
☐	☐	☐
☐	☐	☐
☐	☐	☐
Poor		

JULY 3, DAY OF THE WEEK   S   M   T   W   TH   F   S

MOOD	VIGOR	SLEEP
Excellent		
☐	☐	☐
☐	☐	☐
☐	☐	☐
Poor		

The noise level in some restaurants can reach as high as 110 decibels, which is like trying to dine while running a power chain saw. Eat only at restaurants at which you can feel relaxed. You'll eat more slowly and won't be as likely to overeat—and you'll enjoy your meal a lot more, too.

JULY 4, DAY OF THE WEEK   S   M   T   W   TH   F   S

MOOD	VIGOR	SLEEP
Excellent		
☐	☐	☐
☐	☐	☐
☐	☐	☐
Poor		

JULY 5, DAY OF THE WEEK   S   M   T   W   TH   F   S

MOOD	VIGOR	SLEEP
Excellent		
☐	☐	☐
☐	☐	☐
☐	☐	☐
Poor		

JULY 6, DAY OF THE WEEK   S   M   T   W   TH   F   S

MOOD	VIGOR	SLEEP
Excellent		
☐	☐	☐
☐	☐	☐
☐	☐	☐
Poor		

JULY 7, DAY OF THE WEEK   S   M   T   W   TH   F   S

MOOD	VIGOR	SLEEP
Excellent		
☐	☐	☐
☐	☐	☐
☐	☐	☐
Poor		

July 1–7

NUTRITION LOG

GOALS (# SERVINGS)	WHOLE GRAINS	FRUITS	VEGETABLES	PROTEIN	DAIRY	EXTRAS
	3+	2+	3+	2–4	2–3	VARIABLE
JULY 1	☐	☐	☐	☐	☐	☐
NOTES:						
JULY 2	☐	☐	☐	☐	☐	☐
NOTES:						
JULY 3	☐	☐	☐	☐	☐	☐
NOTES:						
JULY 4	☐	☐	☐	☐	☐	☐
NOTES:						
JULY 5	☐	☐	☐	☐	☐	☐
NOTES:						
JULY 6	☐	☐	☐	☐	☐	☐
NOTES:						
JULY 7	☐	☐	☐	☐	☐	☐
NOTES:						

CALCIUM + VITAMIN D ☐　VITAMIN E ☐　MULTIVITAMIN/MINERAL ☐

PLENTY OF FLUIDS ☐　OTHER SUPPLEMENTS _____

OVERALL COMMENTS

PHYSICAL ACTIVITY

planned, sport, leisure, errands, play
Goal: 30 to 60 minutes most days of the week

DAY	ACTIVITY	TIME

STRENGTH TRAINING

Goal: 2 to 3 times per week

EXERCISE 2 SETS/8 TO 10 REPS	DAY: POUNDS OR ✓	DAY: POUNDS OR ✓	DAY: POUNDS OR ✓

NUMBER OF STEPS

JULY 1	JULY 2	JULY 3	JULY 4	JULY 5	JULY 6	JULY 7

JULY 8–14

When I was a kid, I was always outside running around. I'd play baseball, basketball, or football with the boys. I'd ride my bike or see how fast I could run to school. This was the '60s, when active girls were called tomboys. I don't play much baseball, basketball, or football these days. I do weight training and spend most of my time on the golf course. I still hear, "You hit the ball pretty good for a girl," but they don't call me a tomboy anymore. I guess that's "progress."
We women need to show others that being strong is normal. Our contributions shouldn't be labeled "pretty good for a girl."—BEV

PERSONAL NOTES

JULY 8, DAY OF THE WEEK S M T W TH F S

MOOD	VIGOR	SLEEP
Excellent		
☐	☐	☐
☐	☐	☐
☐	☐	☐
Poor		

JULY 9, DAY OF THE WEEK S M T W TH F S

MOOD	VIGOR	SLEEP
Excellent		
☐	☐	☐
☐	☐	☐
☐	☐	☐
Poor		

JULY 10, DAY OF THE WEEK S M T W TH F S

MOOD	VIGOR	SLEEP
Excellent		
☐	☐	☐
☐	☐	☐
☐	☐	☐
Poor		

Chayote, an exotic vegetable from Latin America with a mild taste like zucchini yet also with a hint of citrus, is a good source of vitamin C and has only 19 calories per serving. Try baking it stuffed with a little cheese, although it can also be eaten raw. (It doesn't even have to be peeled.)

JULY 11, DAY OF THE WEEK   S   M   T   W   TH   F   S

MOOD	VIGOR	SLEEP
Excellent		
☐	☐	☐
☐	☐	☐
☐	☐	☐
Poor		

JULY 12, DAY OF THE WEEK   S   M   T   W   TH   F   S

MOOD	VIGOR	SLEEP
Excellent		
☐	☐	☐
☐	☐	☐
☐	☐	☐
Poor		

JULY 13, DAY OF THE WEEK   S   M   T   W   TH   F   S

MOOD	VIGOR	SLEEP
Excellent		
☐	☐	☐
☐	☐	☐
☐	☐	☐
Poor		

JULY 14, DAY OF THE WEEK   S   M   T   W   TH   F   S

MOOD	VIGOR	SLEEP
Excellent		
☐	☐	☐
☐	☐	☐
☐	☐	☐
Poor		

JULY 8–14
NUTRITION LOG

GOALS (# SERVINGS)	WHOLE GRAINS	FRUITS	VEGETABLES	PROTEIN	DAIRY	EXTRAS
	3+	2+	3+	2–4	2–3	VARIABLE
JULY 8	☐	☐	☐	☐	☐	☐
NOTES:						
JULY 9	☐	☐	☐	☐	☐	☐
NOTES:						
JULY 10	☐	☐	☐	☐	☐	☐
NOTES:						
JULY 11	☐	☐	☐	☐	☐	☐
NOTES:						
JULY 12	☐	☐	☐	☐	☐	☐
NOTES:						
JULY 13	☐	☐	☐	☐	☐	☐
NOTES:						
JULY 14	☐	☐	☐	☐	☐	☐
NOTES:						

CALCIUM + VITAMIN D ☐ **VITAMIN E** ☐ **MULTIVITAMIN/MINERAL** ☐

PLENTY OF FLUIDS ☐ **OTHER SUPPLEMENTS** _____

OVERALL COMMENTS

PHYSICAL ACTIVITY

planned, sport, leisure, errands, play
Goal: 30 to 60 minutes most days of the week

DAY	ACTIVITY	TIME

STRENGTH TRAINING

Goal: 2 to 3 times per week

EXERCISE 2 SETS/8 TO 10 REPS	DAY: POUNDS OR ✓	DAY: POUNDS OR ✓	DAY: POUNDS OR ✓

NUMBER OF STEPS

JULY 8	JULY 9	JULY 10	JULY 11	JULY 12	JULY 13	JULY 14

JULY 15-21

You have to make the very best out of the situation that you find yourself in. This attitude helped me get through a very stressful period recently, when I found myself in a situation where I might have lost my job due to budget cuts. I had just moved to another state to take this job and had no professional contacts in the area. Instead of worrying, I decided I would tell my supervisors that I had not been completely content during my three months on the job and that if they decided to keep me, it would be with the understanding that we'd work together to improve my situation so I could live up to my potential as an employee. Instead of laying me off, they did indeed improve my working conditions. I also used the impending layoffs as motivation to look into a teaching career, something I am now pursuing as a future goal.—JILL

PERSONAL NOTES

JULY 15, DAY OF THE WEEK S   M   T   W   TH   F   S

MOOD	VIGOR	SLEEP
Excellent		
☐	☐	☐
☐	☐	☐
☐	☐	☐
Poor		

JULY 16, DAY OF THE WEEK S   M   T   W   TH   F   S

MOOD	VIGOR	SLEEP
Excellent		
☐	☐	☐
☐	☐	☐
☐	☐	☐
Poor		

JULY 17, DAY OF THE WEEK S   M   T   W   TH   F   S

MOOD	VIGOR	SLEEP
Excellent		
☐	☐	☐
☐	☐	☐
☐	☐	☐
Poor		

Portion sizes are getting larger than ever. Consider that *The Joy of Cooking*'s brownie recipe is exactly the same as it was in the 1960s. But the latest edition says the yield is 16 brownies instead of the original 30, meaning that each brownie is essentially twice as big, point out researchers at New York University. To get a feel for how much you're eating, portion out some foods with measuring cups and spoons. A cup of pasta is two servings, but that's not much pasta—just 64 strands of spaghetti. Measuring out your foods for a couple of days will really help you control your portions and calories.

JULY 18, DAY OF THE WEEK   S   M   T   W   TH   F   S

MOOD	VIGOR	SLEEP
Excellent		
☐	☐	☐
☐	☐	☐
☐	☐	☐
Poor		

JULY 19, DAY OF THE WEEK   S   M   T   W   TH   F   S

MOOD	VIGOR	SLEEP
Excellent		
☐	☐	☐
☐	☐	☐
☐	☐	☐
Poor		

JULY 20, DAY OF THE WEEK   S   M   T   W   TH   F   S

MOOD	VIGOR	SLEEP
Excellent		
☐	☐	☐
☐	☐	☐
☐	☐	☐
Poor		

JULY 21, DAY OF THE WEEK   S   M   T   W   TH   F   S

MOOD	VIGOR	SLEEP
Excellent		
☐	☐	☐
☐	☐	☐
☐	☐	☐
Poor		

July 15–21
NUTRITION LOG

GOALS (# SERVINGS)	WHOLE GRAINS 3+	FRUITS 2+	VEGETABLES 3+	PROTEIN 2–4	DAIRY 2–3	EXTRAS VARIABLE
JULY 15 **NOTES:**	☐	☐	☐	☐	☐	☐
JULY 16 **NOTES:**	☐	☐	☐	☐	☐	☐
JULY 17 **NOTES:**	☐	☐	☐	☐	☐	☐
JULY 18 **NOTES:**	☐	☐	☐	☐	☐	☐
JULY 19 **NOTES:**	☐	☐	☐	☐	☐	☐
JULY 20 **NOTES:**	☐	☐	☐	☐	☐	☐
JULY 21 **NOTES:**	☐	☐	☐	☐	☐	☐

CALCIUM + VITAMIN D ☐ **VITAMIN E** ☐ **MULTIVITAMIN/MINERAL** ☐

PLENTY OF FLUIDS ☐ **OTHER SUPPLEMENTS** _____

OVERALL COMMENTS

PHYSICAL ACTIVITY

planned, sport, leisure, errands, play
Goal: 30 to 60 minutes most days of the week

DAY	ACTIVITY	TIME

STRENGTH TRAINING

Goal: 2 to 3 times per week

EXERCISE 2 SETS/8 TO 10 REPS	DAY: POUNDS OR ✓	DAY: POUNDS OR ✓	DAY: POUNDS OR ✓

NUMBER OF STEPS

JULY 15	JULY 16	JULY 17	JULY 18	JULY 19	JULY 20	JULY 21

JULY 22–28

The British and their stiff upper lip aren't completely off base. When life deals you blows, you just tuck and roll—but make sure you spring right back on your feet. Don't wallow in your misery. Misery passes. Don't feed it. Otherwise, it is like a stray animal—it won't go away because it thinks you like it. I wish I could tell this to everyone who has ever gone through a time of desperate despair. A year from now you will NOT feel this way.—LORI

PERSONAL NOTES

JULY 22, DAY OF THE WEEK   S   M   T   W   TH   F   S

MOOD	VIGOR	SLEEP
Excellent		
☐	☐	☐
☐	☐	☐
☐	☐	☐
Poor		

JULY 23, DAY OF THE WEEK   S   M   T   W   TH   F   S

MOOD	VIGOR	SLEEP
Excellent		
☐	☐	☐
☐	☐	☐
☐	☐	☐
Poor		

JULY 24, DAY OF THE WEEK   S   M   T   W   TH   F   S

MOOD	VIGOR	SLEEP
Excellent		
☐	☐	☐
☐	☐	☐
☐	☐	☐
Poor		

Gardening can be a great workout, as long as it's more strenuous than watering the window boxes. It has been linked with a reduced risk for osteoporosis as well as weight control. Mowing with a power mower for 30 minutes burns 200 calories in a 150-pound person.

JULY 25, DAY OF THE WEEK S M T W TH F S

MOOD	VIGOR	SLEEP
Excellent		
☐	☐	☐
☐	☐	☐
☐	☐	☐
Poor		

JULY 26, DAY OF THE WEEK S M T W TH F S

MOOD	VIGOR	SLEEP
Excellent		
☐	☐	☐
☐	☐	☐
☐	☐	☐
Poor		

JULY 27, DAY OF THE WEEK S M T W TH F S

MOOD	VIGOR	SLEEP
Excellent		
☐	☐	☐
☐	☐	☐
☐	☐	☐
Poor		

JULY 28, DAY OF THE WEEK S M T W TH F S

MOOD	VIGOR	SLEEP
Excellent		
☐	☐	☐
☐	☐	☐
☐	☐	☐
Poor		

July 22–28
Nutrition Log

GOALS (# SERVINGS)	WHOLE GRAINS 3+	FRUITS 2+	VEGETABLES 3+	PROTEIN 2–4	DAIRY 2–3	EXTRAS VARIABLE
JULY 22 NOTES:	☐	☐	☐	☐	☐	☐
JULY 23 NOTES:	☐	☐	☐	☐	☐	☐
JULY 24 NOTES:	☐	☐	☐	☐	☐	☐
JULY 25 NOTES:	☐	☐	☐	☐	☐	☐
JULY 26 NOTES:	☐	☐	☐	☐	☐	☐
JULY 27 NOTES:	☐	☐	☐	☐	☐	☐
JULY 28 NOTES:	☐	☐	☐	☐	☐	☐

CALCIUM + VITAMIN D ☐ **VITAMIN E** ☐ **MULTIVITAMIN/MINERAL** ☐

PLENTY OF FLUIDS ☐ **OTHER SUPPLEMENTS** _____

OVERALL COMMENTS

PHYSICAL ACTIVITY

planned, sport, leisure, errands, play
Goal: 30 to 60 minutes most days of the week

DAY	ACTIVITY	TIME

STRENGTH TRAINING

Goal: 2 to 3 times per week

EXERCISE 2 SETS/8 TO 10 REPS	DAY: POUNDS OR ✓	DAY: POUNDS OR ✓	DAY: POUNDS OR ✓

NUMBER OF STEPS

JULY 22	JULY 23	JULY 24	JULY 25	JULY 26	JULY 27	JULY 28

July 29–31

Personal Notes

JULY 29, DAY OF THE WEEK S   M   T   W   TH   F   S

MOOD	VIGOR	SLEEP
	Excellent	
☐	☐	☐
☐	☐	☐
☐	☐	☐
	Poor	

JULY 30, DAY OF THE WEEK S   M   T   W   TH   F   S

MOOD	VIGOR	SLEEP
	Excellent	
☐	☐	☐
☐	☐	☐
☐	☐	☐
	Poor	

JULY 31, DAY OF THE WEEK S   M   T   W   TH   F   S

MOOD	VIGOR	SLEEP
	Excellent	
☐	☐	☐
☐	☐	☐
☐	☐	☐
	Poor	

JULY 29–31
NUTRITION LOG

GOALS (# SERVINGS)	WHOLE GRAINS	FRUITS	VEGETABLES	PROTEIN	DAIRY	EXTRAS
	3+	2+	3+	2–4	2–3	VARIABLE
JULY 29	☐	☐	☐	☐	☐	☐
NOTES:						
JULY 30	☐	☐	☐	☐	☐	☐
NOTES:						
JULY 31	☐	☐	☐	☐	☐	☐
NOTES:						

CALCIUM + VITAMIN D ☐ VITAMIN E ☐ MULTIVITAMIN/MINERAL ☐

PLENTY OF FLUIDS ☐ OTHER SUPPLEMENTS _____

OVERALL COMMENTS

PHYSICAL ACTIVITY

planned, sport, leisure, errands, play
Goal: 30 to 60 minutes most days of the week

DAY	ACTIVITY	TIME

STRENGTH TRAINING

Goal: 2 to 3 times per week

EXERCISE 2 SETS/8 TO 10 REPS	DAY: POUNDS OR ✓	DAY: POUNDS OR ✓	DAY: POUNDS OR ✓

NUMBER OF STEPS

JULY 29   JULY 30   JULY 31

_____   _____   _____

JULY REVIEW

BRIGHT SPOTS:

_____

GREATEST CHALLENGES:

_____

_____

PATTERNS OBSERVED:

_____

IDENTIFY BARRIERS TO CHANGE AND HOW I AM GOING TO OVERCOME THEM:

PERSONAL

_____

_____

PROFESSIONAL

_____

_____

PERSONAL CARE ATTENTION (flossing teeth, skin care, cutting/coloring hair, etc.):

_____

_____

WELLNESS CHECK (Did I have any sick days?):

_____

_____

BODY WEIGHT: MONTHLY CYCLE DATES (if applicable):

_____

DOCTOR/DENTIST APPOINTMENTS:

_____

_____

MEDICATIONS TAKEN:

_____

_____

_____

Don't Be Myopic

"How many grams of fat are in a half-ounce of potato chips?" "If I eat a slice of pizza, am I getting enough lycopene from the tomato sauce?" "Is it better to have blueberries or raspberries?" I have heard so many people talk about their diets with such grave concern over the smallest details that they run the risk of sucking all the joy out of their own eating. Yes, what you eat is important, and nutrition knowledge is good for tweaking an eating plan. But making the right choices isn't torturous if you keep your eye on the big picture. That is, before worrying about which berries you sprinkle over your yogurt or cereal, ask yourself whether you make sure to include a variety of fruit with your meals and snacks every day. Infinitely more important than whether your pizza sauce has the right amount of a single chemical out of thousands in food is whether you have a salad with two slices of pizza or eat three slices with no vegetable.

Myopia doesn't only express itself as overwrought concern. It can also be manifested as a kind of blind smugness. Consider the person who won't *touch* red meat, which happens to have some essential minerals in short supply in women's diets, but will down a half pint of super-premium ice cream, which has as much saturated fat as the meat but also much more sugar and much less of some key nutrients.

In the exercise realm, myopia tends to be exhibited in concerns over what's the *best* exercise, the *most* effective move, and so on. The best exercise, even if it doesn't work your body as well as some others, is the one you enjoy and will stick with.

In other words, relax—and concentrate on the big picture. Focus on whether you're eating right in general and getting the appropriate amount of physical activity, and the rest will fall into place.

August

August 1–7

I had already been participating in the Strong Women *program when I convinced my administrator to bring in a local yoga instructor at the workplace. Each week, people who passed in the hallway but didn't know each other participated in learning this new skill. Now, when we see each other, it's a reminder of the peaceful environment where we first truly "met." It calms me right down, even though it's a very subtle cue.*—Marian

Personal Notes

AUGUST 1, DAY OF THE WEEK   S   M   T   W   TH   F   S

MOOD	VIGOR	SLEEP
	Excellent	
☐	☐	☐
☐	☐	☐
☐	☐	☐
	Poor	

AUGUST 2, DAY OF THE WEEK   S   M   T   W   TH   F   S

MOOD	VIGOR	SLEEP
	Excellent	
☐	☐	☐
☐	☐	☐
☐	☐	☐
	Poor	

AUGUST 3, DAY OF THE WEEK   S   M   T   W   TH   F   S

MOOD	VIGOR	SLEEP
	Excellent	
☐	☐	☐
☐	☐	☐
☐	☐	☐
	Poor	

Keep your free weights in a canvas bag right in the room where you plan to lift weights. Even having to retrieve your weights from another room can weaken resolve if you're not in the mood to strength train. If you exercise at the gym, place your workout bag at the door the night before to goad you into going the next day.

AUGUST 4, DAY OF THE WEEK   S   M   T   W   TH   F   S

MOOD	VIGOR	SLEEP
Excellent		
☐	☐	☐
☐	☐	☐
☐	☐	☐
Poor		

AUGUST 5, DAY OF THE WEEK   S   M   T   W   TH   F   S

MOOD	VIGOR	SLEEP
Excellent		
☐	☐	☐
☐	☐	☐
☐	☐	☐
Poor		

AUGUST 6, DAY OF THE WEEK   S   M   T   W   TH   F   S

MOOD	VIGOR	SLEEP
Excellent		
☐	☐	☐
☐	☐	☐
☐	☐	☐
Poor		

AUGUST 7, DAY OF THE WEEK   S   M   T   W   TH   F   S

MOOD	VIGOR	SLEEP
Excellent		
☐	☐	☐
☐	☐	☐
☐	☐	☐
Poor		

AUGUST 1–7
NUTRITION LOG

GOALS (# SERVINGS)	WHOLE GRAINS 3+	FRUITS 2+	VEGETABLES 3+	PROTEIN 2–4	DAIRY 2–3	EXTRAS VARIABLE
AUGUST 1	☐	☐	☐	☐	☐	☐
NOTES:						
AUGUST 2	☐	☐	☐	☐	☐	☐
NOTES:						
AUGUST 3	☐	☐	☐	☐	☐	☐
NOTES:						
AUGUST 4	☐	☐	☐	☐	☐	☐
NOTES:						
AUGUST 5	☐	☐	☐	☐	☐	☐
NOTES:						
AUGUST 6	☐	☐	☐	☐	☐	☐
NOTES:						
AUGUST 7	☐	☐	☐	☐	☐	☐
NOTES:						

CALCIUM + VITAMIN D ☐ **VITAMIN E** ☐ **MULTIVITAMIN/MINERAL** ☐

PLENTY OF FLUIDS ☐ **OTHER SUPPLEMENTS** _____

OVERALL COMMENTS

PHYSICAL ACTIVITY

planned, sport, leisure, errands, play
Goal: 30 to 60 minutes most days of the week

DAY	ACTIVITY	TIME

STRENGTH TRAINING

Goal: 2 to 3 times per week

EXERCISE 2 SETS/8 TO 10 REPS	DAY: POUNDS OR ✓	DAY: POUNDS OR ✓	DAY: POUNDS OR ✓

NUMBER OF STEPS

AUGUST 1   AUGUST 2   AUGUST 3   AUGUST 4   AUGUST 5   AUGUST 6   AUGUST 7

_____   _____   _____   _____   _____   _____   _____

August 8–14

I take a cardio-kickboxing class three to five times a week. Regular exercise not only helps to keep me in shape, but it's also an effective stress reliever. If I've had a particularly frustrating workday or I'm grappling with a personal problem, I can easily (and harmlessly) vent by punching or kicking the hell out of a bag. While it doesn't change the way my day went or solve any problems, it still makes me feel better. I'm the oldest person in the class by about 25 years and undoubtedly the only one who's menopausal. And while I find the differences between me and my youthful classmates daunting at times, we share a lot of camaraderie as well.—Bernadette

Personal Notes

AUGUST 8, DAY OF THE WEEK   S   M   T   W   TH   F   S

MOOD	VIGOR	SLEEP
Excellent		
☐	☐	☐
☐	☐	☐
☐	☐	☐
Poor		

AUGUST 9, DAY OF THE WEEK   S   M   T   W   TH   F   S

MOOD	VIGOR	SLEEP
Excellent		
☐	☐	☐
☐	☐	☐
☐	☐	☐
Poor		

AUGUST 10, DAY OF THE WEEK   S   M   T   W   TH   F   S

MOOD	VIGOR	SLEEP
Excellent		
☐	☐	☐
☐	☐	☐
☐	☐	☐
Poor		

Tired of potatoes and rice as your dinner starches? Try a barley pilaf for both its whole-grain benefits and delicious taste. Sauté some chopped onion in a little bit of oil, then add a cup of barley (which you'll find in the rice aisle) and stir. Add 1¾ cups canned vegetable or chicken broth and let simmer, covered, for about 20 minutes. It's done when the water's gone, just like rice. You'll get about four servings.

AUGUST 11, DAY OF THE WEEK   S   M   T   W   TH   F   S

MOOD	VIGOR	SLEEP
Excellent		
☐	☐	☐
☐	☐	☐
☐	☐	☐
Poor		

AUGUST 12, DAY OF THE WEEK   S   M   T   W   TH   F   S

MOOD	VIGOR	SLEEP
Excellent		
☐	☐	☐
☐	☐	☐
☐	☐	☐
Poor		

AUGUST 13, DAY OF THE WEEK   S   M   T   W   TH   F   S

MOOD	VIGOR	SLEEP
Excellent		
☐	☐	☐
☐	☐	☐
☐	☐	☐
Poor		

AUGUST 14, DAY OF THE WEEK   S   M   T   W   TH   F   S

MOOD	VIGOR	SLEEP
Excellent		
☐	☐	☐
☐	☐	☐
☐	☐	☐
Poor		

AUGUST 8–14
NUTRITION LOG

	WHOLE GRAINS	FRUITS	VEGETABLES	PROTEIN	DAIRY	EXTRAS
GOALS (# SERVINGS)	3+	2+	3+	2–4	2–3	VARIABLE
AUGUST 8	☐	☐	☐	☐	☐	☐
NOTES:						
AUGUST 9	☐	☐	☐	☐	☐	☐
NOTES:						
AUGUST 10	☐	☐	☐	☐	☐	☐
NOTES:						
AUGUST 11	☐	☐	☐	☐	☐	☐
NOTES:						
AUGUST 12	☐	☐	☐	☐	☐	☐
NOTES:						
AUGUST 13	☐	☐	☐	☐	☐	☐
NOTES:						
AUGUST 14	☐	☐	☐	☐	☐	☐
NOTES:						

CALCIUM + VITAMIN D ☐ **VITAMIN E** ☐ **MULTIVITAMIN/MINERAL** ☐

PLENTY OF FLUIDS ☐ **OTHER SUPPLEMENTS** _____

OVERALL COMMENTS

PHYSICAL ACTIVITY

planned, sport, leisure, errands, play
Goal: 30 to 60 minutes most days of the week

DAY	ACTIVITY	TIME

STRENGTH TRAINING

Goal: 2 to 3 times per week

EXERCISE 2 SETS/8 TO 10 REPS	DAY: POUNDS OR ✓	DAY: POUNDS OR ✓	DAY: POUNDS OR ✓

NUMBER OF STEPS

AUGUST 8	AUGUST 9	AUGUST 10	AUGUST 11	AUGUST 12	AUGUST 13	AUGUST 14

AUGUST 15–21

I work for a nonprofit affordable housing organization, and I often find it difficult to leave my work at the office. But there are nights now and then when I feel the sudden need to close out everything and look within. When this happens, I turn out all the lights, light a candle or two, run a bath, turn on soothing music, turn off the phone, and let my harried thoughts slip away, releasing myself from my burdens one by one. It may take a while, but I try to spend some long moments imagining myself wrapped in kindness and serenity. I breathe, I listen to the crickets outside my window, and I remember that what is most important is to feel connected to life, to live as though I have a place in the world. I make room in my mind for loving thoughts about myself and loved ones, knowing that, with good practice in moments of meditation like this one, I can remember to extend that love outward to the world. Awareness of purpose is a circle that regenerates itself. I look within so that I can be stronger to act without.—ELIN

PERSONAL NOTES

AUGUST 15, DAY OF THE WEEK   S   M   T   W   TH   F   S

	MOOD	VIGOR	SLEEP
		Excellent	
	☐	☐	☐
	☐	☐	☐
	☐	☐	☐
		Poor	

AUGUST 16, DAY OF THE WEEK   S   M   T   W   TH   F   S

	MOOD	VIGOR	SLEEP
		Excellent	
	☐	☐	☐
	☐	☐	☐
	☐	☐	☐
		Poor	

AUGUST 17, DAY OF THE WEEK   S   M   T   W   TH   F   S

	MOOD	VIGOR	SLEEP
		Excellent	
	☐	☐	☐
	☐	☐	☐
	☐	☐	☐
		Poor	

Always lift a weight through the full range of motion. For example, a common mistake people make when doing the knee extension is to extend the knee only part way out. To get the full benefit to your knee joint and quadriceps muscles, work on extending your leg completely. If you have knee problems, increase your range of motion slowly from one exercise session to the next. Over a couple of months, your legs will be stronger and your knees more flexible.

AUGUST 18, DAY OF THE WEEK   S   M   T   W   TH   F   S

MOOD	VIGOR	SLEEP
Excellent		
☐	☐	☐
☐	☐	☐
☐	☐	☐
Poor		

AUGUST 19, DAY OF THE WEEK   S   M   T   W   TH   F   S

MOOD	VIGOR	SLEEP
Excellent		
☐	☐	☐
☐	☐	☐
☐	☐	☐
Poor		

AUGUST 20, DAY OF THE WEEK   S   M   T   W   TH   F   S

MOOD	VIGOR	SLEEP
Excellent		
☐	☐	☐
☐	☐	☐
☐	☐	☐
Poor		

AUGUST 21, DAY OF THE WEEK   S   M   T   W   TH   F   S

MOOD	VIGOR	SLEEP
Excellent		
☐	☐	☐
☐	☐	☐
☐	☐	☐
Poor		

AUGUST 15–21
NUTRITION LOG

GOALS (# SERVINGS)	WHOLE GRAINS 3+	FRUITS 2+	VEGETABLES 3+	PROTEIN 2–4	DAIRY 2–3	EXTRAS VARIABLE
AUGUST 15	☐	☐	☐	☐	☐	☐
NOTES:						
AUGUST 16	☐	☐	☐	☐	☐	☐
NOTES:						
AUGUST 17	☐	☐	☐	☐	☐	☐
NOTES:						
AUGUST 18	☐	☐	☐	☐	☐	☐
NOTES:						
AUGUST 19	☐	☐	☐	☐	☐	☐
NOTES:						
AUGUST 20	☐	☐	☐	☐	☐	☐
NOTES:						
AUGUST 21	☐	☐	☐	☐	☐	☐
NOTES:						

CALCIUM + VITAMIN D ☐ VITAMIN E ☐ MULTIVITAMIN/MINERAL ☐

PLENTY OF FLUIDS ☐ OTHER SUPPLEMENTS _____

OVERALL COMMENTS

PHYSICAL ACTIVITY

planned, sport, leisure, errands, play
Goal: 30 to 60 minutes most days of the week

DAY	ACTIVITY	TIME

STRENGTH TRAINING

Goal: 2 to 3 times per week

EXERCISE 2 SETS/8 TO 10 REPS	DAY: POUNDS OR ✓	DAY: POUNDS OR ✓	DAY: POUNDS OR ✓

NUMBER OF STEPS

AUGUST 15	AUGUST 16	AUGUST 17	AUGUST 18	AUGUST 19	AUGUST 20	AUGUST 21

AUGUST 22–28

I am aware that I am by no means Super Woman, so on the days that I cannot handle the gym, I round up some of my best venting buddies and off we go for some unhealthy margaritas and some healthy bitching.—SKYE

PERSONAL NOTES

AUGUST 22, DAY OF THE WEEK   S   M   T   W   TH   F   S

MOOD	VIGOR	SLEEP
Excellent		
☐	☐	☐
☐	☐	☐
☐	☐	☐
Poor		

AUGUST 23, DAY OF THE WEEK   S   M   T   W   TH   F   S

MOOD	VIGOR	SLEEP
Excellent		
☐	☐	☐
☐	☐	☐
☐	☐	☐
Poor		

AUGUST 24, DAY OF THE WEEK   S   M   T   W   TH   F   S

MOOD	VIGOR	SLEEP
Excellent		
☐	☐	☐
☐	☐	☐
☐	☐	☐
Poor		

Here's the easiest peach sorbet in the world. Freeze a can of peaches (in heavy syrup) for 18 hours. After freezing, submerge the can in hot water for a minute or so, open it, and cut the frozen product into 1-inch slices. Then pulse the peaches and syrup in a food processor until smooth. A half-cup serving contains 100 calories.

AUGUST 25, DAY OF THE WEEK   S   M   T   W   TH   F   S

	MOOD	VIGOR	SLEEP
Excellent			
	☐	☐	☐
	☐	☐	☐
	☐	☐	☐
Poor			

AUGUST 26, DAY OF THE WEEK   S   M   T   W   TH   F   S

	MOOD	VIGOR	SLEEP
Excellent			
	☐	☐	☐
	☐	☐	☐
	☐	☐	☐
Poor			

AUGUST 27, DAY OF THE WEEK   S   M   T   W   TH   F   S

	MOOD	VIGOR	SLEEP
Excellent			
	☐	☐	☐
	☐	☐	☐
	☐	☐	☐
Poor			

AUGUST 28, DAY OF THE WEEK   S   M   T   W   TH   F   S

	MOOD	VIGOR	SLEEP
Excellent			
	☐	☐	☐
	☐	☐	☐
	☐	☐	☐
Poor			

AUGUST 22–28
NUTRITION LOG

	WHOLE GRAINS	FRUITS	VEGETABLES	PROTEIN	DAIRY	EXTRAS
GOALS (# SERVINGS)	3+	2+	3+	2–4	2–3	VARIABLE
AUGUST 22	☐	☐	☐	☐	☐	☐
NOTES:						
AUGUST 23	☐	☐	☐	☐	☐	☐
NOTES:						
AUGUST 24	☐	☐	☐	☐	☐	☐
NOTES:						
AUGUST 25	☐	☐	☐	☐	☐	☐
NOTES:						
AUGUST 26	☐	☐	☐	☐	☐	☐
NOTES:						
AUGUST 27	☐	☐	☐	☐	☐	☐
NOTES:						
AUGUST 28	☐	☐	☐	☐	☐	☐
NOTES:						

CALCIUM + VITAMIN D ☐ VITAMIN E ☐ MULTIVITAMIN/MINERAL ☐

PLENTY OF FLUIDS ☐ OTHER SUPPLEMENTS _____

OVERALL COMMENTS

PHYSICAL ACTIVITY

planned, sport, leisure, errands, play
Goal: 30 to 60 minutes most days of the week

DAY	ACTIVITY	TIME

STRENGTH TRAINING

Goal: 2 to 3 times per week

EXERCISE 2 SETS/8 TO 10 REPS	DAY: POUNDS OR ✓	DAY: POUNDS OR ✓	DAY: POUNDS OR ✓

NUMBER OF STEPS

AUGUST 22	AUGUST 23	AUGUST 24	AUGUST 25	AUGUST 26	AUGUST 27	AUGUST 28

AUGUST 29–31

PERSONAL NOTES

AUGUST 29, DAY OF THE WEEK   S   M   T   W   TH   F   S

MOOD	VIGOR	SLEEP
	Excellent	
☐	☐	☐
☐	☐	☐
☐	☐	☐
	Poor	

AUGUST 30, DAY OF THE WEEK   S   M   T   W   TH   F   S

MOOD	VIGOR	SLEEP
	Excellent	
☐	☐	☐
☐	☐	☐
☐	☐	☐
	Poor	

AUGUST 31, DAY OF THE WEEK   S   M   T   W   TH   F   S

MOOD	VIGOR	SLEEP
	Excellent	
☐	☐	☐
☐	☐	☐
☐	☐	☐
	Poor	

AUGUST 29–31
NUTRITION LOG

GOALS (# SERVINGS)	WHOLE GRAINS 3+	FRUITS 2+	VEGETABLES 3+	PROTEIN 2–4	DAIRY 2–3	EXTRAS VARIABLE
AUGUST 29 NOTES:	☐	☐	☐	☐	☐	☐
AUGUST 30 NOTES:	☐	☐	☐	☐	☐	☐
AUGUST 31 NOTES:	☐	☐	☐	☐	☐	☐

CALCIUM + VITAMIN D ☐ VITAMIN E ☐ MULTIVITAMIN/MINERAL ☐

PLENTY OF FLUIDS ☐ OTHER SUPPLEMENTS _____

OVERALL COMMENTS

PHYSICAL ACTIVITY

planned, sport, leisure, errands, play
Goal: 30 to 60 minutes most days of the week

DAY	ACTIVITY	TIME

STRENGTH TRAINING

Goal: 2 to 3 times per week

EXERCISE 2 SETS/8 TO 10 REPS	DAY: POUNDS OR ✓	DAY: POUNDS OR ✓	DAY: POUNDS OR ✓

NUMBER OF STEPS

AUGUST 29   AUGUST 30   AUGUST 31

_____   _____   _____

AUGUST REVIEW

BRIGHT SPOTS:
_____

GREATEST CHALLENGES:
_____
_____
_____

PATTERNS OBSERVED:
_____
_____

IDENTIFY BARRIERS TO CHANGE AND HOW I AM GOING TO OVERCOME THEM:

    PERSONAL
_____
_____

    PROFESSIONAL
_____
_____

PERSONAL CARE ATTENTION (flossing teeth, skin care, cutting/coloring hair, etc.):
_____
_____

WELLNESS CHECK (Did I have any sick days?):
_____
_____

BODY WEIGHT: MONTHLY CYCLE DATES (if applicable):
_____

DOCTOR/DENTIST APPOINTMENTS:
_____
_____

MEDICATIONS TAKEN:
_____
_____
_____

Take a Deep Breath

Several years ago I started to experience something very strange (although I have since heard from other women that the same thing happened to them). I would be driving somewhere on the highway and have a complete brain blankout. I don't mean I stopped being able to drive—that came automatically, so I wasn't in danger. But for 45 seconds or so I truly could not figure out where I was. I had lost all orientation.

After about four episodes of this, I went to the doctor. He asked me what was going on in my life. I told him, with some prompting on his part, that I was still nursing, had two other children under the age of four, a full-time job, a research report due, teaching responsibilities, and was soon going to be moving to a new house—but that "everything was just fine." Of course, as I recited my litany of responsibilities, I was able to see what the problem was. I was on stress overload.

Just holding that knowledge in my hand helped me a great deal. While I couldn't shirk any of my duties, I started a routine of taking a longer shower in the evening and, during that time, trying to clear my head and totally relax. I also learned back then to close my office door at least once a day and just sit for a few minutes without thinking about anything. That is, I learned to elicit the relaxation response—a meditative state where you get in touch with your body by emptying your brain.

Taking these moments for myself is most important for me in September, my most stressful month. My kids are getting back on a tight schedule with school and, as an academic, so am I. Learning that stress is a part of life but that you can steal moments for yourself to take a deep breath has really helped me.

September

SEPTEMBER 1–7

One of my favorite authors observed, "Argue for your limitations and they are yours." I remember this whenever I start to think, "I can't." Facing fear goes a long way toward reducing the barriers. I learned to ride a bicycle at the age of 49, and the next year put more than 500 miles on it. I found a great joy in that year. The wonder of being so strong and feeling so capable made riding become a kind of physical meditation that translated to the emotional. I found old problems quietly solved themselves, with solutions seeming obvious. As the cyclists say, "The hills flatten out as we get stronger." Facing down fear makes all problems smaller and more manageable.—CYNTHIA

PERSONAL NOTES

SEPTEMBER 1, DAY OF THE WEEK   S   M   T   W   TH   F   S

MOOD	VIGOR	SLEEP
	Excellent	
☐	☐	☐
☐	☐	☐
☐	☐	☐
	Poor	

SEPTEMBER 2, DAY OF THE WEEK   S   M   T   W   TH   F   S

MOOD	VIGOR	SLEEP
	Excellent	
☐	☐	☐
☐	☐	☐
☐	☐	☐
	Poor	

SEPTEMBER 3, DAY OF THE WEEK   S   M   T   W   TH   F   S

MOOD	VIGOR	SLEEP
	Excellent	
☐	☐	☐
☐	☐	☐
☐	☐	☐
	Poor	

Tofu is a wonderful protein source that's very low in saturated fat. Firm tofu is great stir-fried with vegetables and teriyaki sauce. Silken tofu is easy to incorporate into meals, too. Add some to scrambled eggs or egg salad; toss some in the blender when making fruit smoothies; or puree some and use it in recipes in place of mayonnaise, sour cream, or cream cheese. You can even freeze silken tofu to get it to the right texture for crumbling into stews and casseroles.

SEPTEMBER 4, DAY OF THE WEEK S M T W TH F S

	MOOD	VIGOR	SLEEP
		Excellent	
	☐	☐	☐
	☐	☐	☐
	☐	☐	☐
		Poor	

SEPTEMBER 5, DAY OF THE WEEK S M T W TH F S

	MOOD	VIGOR	SLEEP
		Excellent	
	☐	☐	☐
	☐	☐	☐
	☐	☐	☐
		Poor	

SEPTEMBER 6, DAY OF THE WEEK S M T W TH F S

	MOOD	VIGOR	SLEEP
		Excellent	
	☐	☐	☐
	☐	☐	☐
	☐	☐	☐
		Poor	

SEPTEMBER 7, DAY OF THE WEEK S M T W TH F S

	MOOD	VIGOR	SLEEP
		Excellent	
	☐	☐	☐
	☐	☐	☐
	☐	☐	☐
		Poor	

SEPTEMBER 1–7
NUTRITION LOG

GOALS (# SERVINGS)	WHOLE GRAINS 3+	FRUITS 2+	VEGETABLES 3+	PROTEIN 2–4	DAIRY 2–3	EXTRAS VARIABLE
SEPTEMBER 1 NOTES:	☐	☐	☐	☐	☐	☐
SEPTEMBER 2 NOTES:	☐	☐	☐	☐	☐	☐
SEPTEMBER 3 NOTES:	☐	☐	☐	☐	☐	☐
SEPTEMBER 4 NOTES:	☐	☐	☐	☐	☐	☐
SEPTEMBER 5 NOTES:	☐	☐	☐	☐	☐	☐
SEPTEMBER 6 NOTES:	☐	☐	☐	☐	☐	☐
SEPTEMBER 7 NOTES:	☐	☐	☐	☐	☐	☐

CALCIUM + VITAMIN D ☐ **VITAMIN E** ☐ **MULTIVITAMIN/MINERAL** ☐

PLENTY OF FLUIDS ☐ **OTHER SUPPLEMENTS** _____

OVERALL COMMENTS

PHYSICAL ACTIVITY

planned, sport, leisure, errands, play
Goal: 30 to 60 minutes most days of the week

DAY	ACTIVITY	TIME

STRENGTH TRAINING

Goal: 2 to 3 times per week

EXERCISE 2 SETS/8 TO 10 REPS	DAY: POUNDS OR ✓	DAY: POUNDS OR ✓	DAY: POUNDS OR ✓

NUMBER OF STEPS

SEPTEMBER 1   SEPTEMBER 2   SEPTEMBER 3   SEPTEMBER 4   SEPTEMBER 5   SEPTEMBER 6   SEPTEMBER 7

_____   _____   _____   _____   _____   _____   _____

SEPTEMBER 8–14

As an overweight child and young adult, I never imagined that running would be such an important part of my life. However, in my mid 20s I took a risk and set out on one of my first "shuffles." I am currently preparing to run my fourth marathon. The benefits—both physical and mental—have been extraordinary. Running calms me and raises my spirits at the same time. After a run I am a more positive person than before I took my first step out the door. I realize that I do have discipline, fitness, and endurance; that I can set a goal and reach it; that I am indeed an athlete.—HELEN

PERSONAL NOTES

SEPTEMBER 8, DAY OF THE WEEK   S   M   T   W   TH   F   S

MOOD	VIGOR	SLEEP
Excellent		
☐	☐	☐
☐	☐	☐
☐	☐	☐
Poor		

SEPTEMBER 9, DAY OF THE WEEK   S   M   T   W   TH   F   S

MOOD	VIGOR	SLEEP
Excellent		
☐	☐	☐
☐	☐	☐
☐	☐	☐
Poor		

SEPTEMBER 10, DAY OF THE WEEK   S   M   T   W   TH   F   S

MOOD	VIGOR	SLEEP
Excellent		
☐	☐	☐
☐	☐	☐
☐	☐	☐
Poor		

Remember, if during strength training you can do more than 15 repetitions with a particular amount of weight, it is time to increase the weight. Ideally, the weight should be heavy enough to make you rest after 8 to 12 repetitions.

SEPTEMBER 11, DAY OF THE WEEK S M T W TH F S

	MOOD	VIGOR	SLEEP
	Excellent		
	☐	☐	☐
	☐	☐	☐
	☐	☐	☐
	Poor		

SEPTEMBER 12, DAY OF THE WEEK S M T W TH F S

	MOOD	VIGOR	SLEEP
	Excellent		
	☐	☐	☐
	☐	☐	☐
	☐	☐	☐
	Poor		

SEPTEMBER 13, DAY OF THE WEEK S M T W TH F S

	MOOD	VIGOR	SLEEP
	Excellent		
	☐	☐	☐
	☐	☐	☐
	☐	☐	☐
	Poor		

SEPTEMBER 14, DAY OF THE WEEK S M T W TH F S

	MOOD	VIGOR	SLEEP
	Excellent		
	☐	☐	☐
	☐	☐	☐
	☐	☐	☐
	Poor		

SEPTEMBER 8–14
NUTRITION LOG

GOALS (# SERVINGS)	WHOLE GRAINS 3+	FRUITS 2+	VEGETABLES 3+	PROTEIN 2–4	DAIRY 2–3	EXTRAS VARIABLE
SEPTEMBER 8	☐	☐	☐	☐	☐	☐
NOTES:						
SEPTEMBER 9	☐	☐	☐	☐	☐	☐
NOTES:						
SEPTEMBER 10	☐	☐	☐	☐	☐	☐
NOTES:						
SEPTEMBER 11	☐	☐	☐	☐	☐	☐
NOTES:						
SEPTEMBER 12	☐	☐	☐	☐	☐	☐
NOTES:						
SEPTEMBER 13	☐	☐	☐	☐	☐	☐
NOTES:						
SEPTEMBER 14	☐	☐	☐	☐	☐	☐
NOTES:						

CALCIUM + VITAMIN D ☐   VITAMIN E ☐   MULTIVITAMIN/MINERAL ☐

PLENTY OF FLUIDS ☐   OTHER SUPPLEMENTS _____

OVERALL COMMENTS

PHYSICAL ACTIVITY

planned, sport, leisure, errands, play
Goal: 30 to 60 minutes most days of the week

DAY	ACTIVITY	TIME

STRENGTH TRAINING

Goal: 2 to 3 times per week

EXERCISE 2 SETS/8 TO 10 REPS	DAY: POUNDS OR ✓	DAY: POUNDS OR ✓	DAY: POUNDS OR ✓

NUMBER OF STEPS

SEPTEMBER 8   SEPTEMBER 9   SEPTEMBER 10   SEPTEMBER 11   SEPTEMBER 12   SEPTEMBER 13   SEPTEMBER 14

_____ _____ _____ _____ _____ _____ _____

SEPTEMBER 15–21

I lost my sight at age 26. No hope of recovery. It was 1985—no such thing yet as the Americans with Disabilities Act. My job went, too. My self-esteem plummeted. And without regular exercise to boost me, I was headed for a crash. A counselor suggested I try a swimming class. The first day, I pushed off the edge and careened from one lane-marker to the other, all the way down and back. "Reach in front of you," the instructor shouted, hoping to teach me to swim straight. "Then pull back toward your belly button." I tried, but in the end I remained an underwater pinball. Still, moving forward in space, running into things yet staying unhurt—it was downright liberating. These days I swim three times a week. When sharing a lane, I stay straight by tapping the lane-marker with every right-hand stroke. It all feels good—so good, in fact, that I've started working again at the local university. My job? Modeling nude for art students.—BETH

PERSONAL NOTES

SEPTEMBER 15, DAY OF THE WEEK   S   M   T   W   TH   F   S

MOOD	VIGOR	SLEEP
Excellent		
☐	☐	☐
☐	☐	☐
☐	☐	☐
Poor		

SEPTEMBER 16, DAY OF THE WEEK   S   M   T   W   TH   F   S

MOOD	VIGOR	SLEEP
Excellent		
☐	☐	☐
☐	☐	☐
☐	☐	☐
Poor		

SEPTEMBER 17, DAY OF THE WEEK   S   M   T   W   TH   F   S

MOOD	VIGOR	SLEEP
Excellent		
☐	☐	☐
☐	☐	☐
☐	☐	☐
Poor		

Turn a whole-wheat wrap into an entrée. Stuff with a cup of cooked broccoli or spinach and a quarter cup of shredded Cheddar cheese, for instance, or a half-cup of salsa and a half-cup of beans. It's instant portion control—a meal for fewer than 300 calories!

SEPTEMBER 18, DAY OF THE WEEK   S   M   T   W   TH   F   S

MOOD	VIGOR	SLEEP
Excellent		
☐	☐	☐
☐	☐	☐
☐	☐	☐
Poor		

SEPTEMBER 19, DAY OF THE WEEK   S   M   T   W   TH   F   S

MOOD	VIGOR	SLEEP
Excellent		
☐	☐	☐
☐	☐	☐
☐	☐	☐
Poor		

SEPTEMBER 20, DAY OF THE WEEK   S   M   T   W   TH   F   S

MOOD	VIGOR	SLEEP
Excellent		
☐	☐	☐
☐	☐	☐
☐	☐	☐
Poor		

SEPTEMBER 21, DAY OF THE WEEK   S   M   T   W   TH   F   S

MOOD	VIGOR	SLEEP
Excellent		
☐	☐	☐
☐	☐	☐
☐	☐	☐
Poor		

SEPTEMBER 15–21
NUTRITION LOG

GOALS (# SERVINGS)	WHOLE GRAINS 3+	FRUITS 2+	VEGETABLES 3+	PROTEIN 2–4	DAIRY 2–3	EXTRAS VARIABLE
SEPTEMBER 15	☐	☐	☐	☐	☐	☐
NOTES:						
SEPTEMBER 16	☐	☐	☐	☐	☐	☐
NOTES:						
SEPTEMBER 17	☐	☐	☐	☐	☐	☐
NOTES:						
SEPTEMBER 18	☐	☐	☐	☐	☐	☐
NOTES:						
SEPTEMBER 19	☐	☐	☐	☐	☐	☐
NOTES:						
SEPTEMBER 20	☐	☐	☐	☐	☐	☐
NOTES:						
SEPTEMBER 21	☐	☐	☐	☐	☐	☐
NOTES:						

CALCIUM + VITAMIN D ☐   VITAMIN E ☐   MULTIVITAMIN/MINERAL ☐

PLENTY OF FLUIDS ☐   OTHER SUPPLEMENTS _____

OVERALL COMMENTS

PHYSICAL ACTIVITY

planned, sport, leisure, errands, play
Goal: 30 to 60 minutes most days of the week

DAY	ACTIVITY	TIME

STRENGTH TRAINING

Goal: 2 to 3 times per week

EXERCISE 2 SETS/8 TO 10 REPS	DAY: POUNDS OR ✓	DAY: POUNDS OR ✓	DAY: POUNDS OR ✓

NUMBER OF STEPS

SEPTEMBER 15 SEPTEMBER 16 SEPTEMBER 17 SEPTEMBER 18 SEPTEMBER 19 SEPTEMBER 20 SEPTEMBER 21

SEPTEMBER 22–28

Someone once posed this question to me: "If you could have a million dollars with the one condition that you could never exercise again, would you take it? Five million? Ten million?" My answer was quick and easy: "No, no, no." It was at that moment that I realized how crucial exercise was to my well-being.—CHRISTINE

PERSONAL NOTES

SEPTEMBER 22, DAY OF THE WEEK   S   M   T   W   TH   F   S

MOOD	VIGOR	SLEEP
Excellent		
☐	☐	☐
☐	☐	☐
☐	☐	☐
Poor		

SEPTEMBER 23, DAY OF THE WEEK   S   M   T   W   TH   F   S

MOOD	VIGOR	SLEEP
Excellent		
☐	☐	☐
☐	☐	☐
☐	☐	☐
Poor		

SEPTEMBER 24, DAY OF THE WEEK   S   M   T   W   TH   F   S

MOOD	VIGOR	SLEEP
Excellent		
☐	☐	☐
☐	☐	☐
☐	☐	☐
Poor		

Whenever you are waiting in line for an elevator or at the grocery store checkout, strengthen your calf muscles—and improve your balance—by doing toe stands. They are so subtle no one will even notice, but you'll get the benefit of better looking calves!

SEPTEMBER 25, DAY OF THE WEEK S M T W TH F S

MOOD	VIGOR	SLEEP
Excellent		
☐	☐	☐
☐	☐	☐
☐	☐	☐
Poor		

SEPTEMBER 26, DAY OF THE WEEK S M T W TH F S

MOOD	VIGOR	SLEEP
Excellent		
☐	☐	☐
☐	☐	☐
☐	☐	☐
Poor		

SEPTEMBER 27, DAY OF THE WEEK S M T W TH F S

MOOD	VIGOR	SLEEP
Excellent		
☐	☐	☐
☐	☐	☐
☐	☐	☐
Poor		

SEPTEMBER 28, DAY OF THE WEEK S M T W TH F S

MOOD	VIGOR	SLEEP
Excellent		
☐	☐	☐
☐	☐	☐
☐	☐	☐
Poor		

SEPTEMBER 22–28
NUTRITION LOG

GOALS (# SERVINGS)	WHOLE GRAINS 3+	FRUITS 2+	VEGETABLES 3+	PROTEIN 2–4	DAIRY 2–3	EXTRAS VARIABLE
SEPTEMBER 22 **NOTES:**	☐	☐	☐	☐	☐	☐
SEPTEMBER 23 **NOTES:**	☐	☐	☐	☐	☐	☐
SEPTEMBER 24 **NOTES:**	☐	☐	☐	☐	☐	☐
SEPTEMBER 25 **NOTES:**	☐	☐	☐	☐	☐	☐
SEPTEMBER 26 **NOTES:**	☐	☐	☐	☐	☐	☐
SEPTEMBER 27 **NOTES:**	☐	☐	☐	☐	☐	☐
SEPTEMBER 28 **NOTES:**	☐	☐	☐	☐	☐	☐

CALCIUM + VITAMIN D ☐ **VITAMIN E** ☐ **MULTIVITAMIN/MINERAL** ☐

PLENTY OF FLUIDS ☐ **OTHER SUPPLEMENTS** _____

OVERALL COMMENTS

PHYSICAL ACTIVITY

planned, sport, leisure, errands, play
Goal: 30 to 60 minutes most days of the week

DAY	ACTIVITY	TIME

STRENGTH TRAINING

Goal: 2 to 3 times per week

EXERCISE 2 SETS/8 TO 10 REPS	DAY: POUNDS OR ✓	DAY: POUNDS OR ✓	DAY: POUNDS OR ✓

NUMBER OF STEPS

SEPTEMBER 22 SEPTEMBER 23 SEPTEMBER 24 SEPTEMBER 25 SEPTEMBER 26 SEPTEMBER 27 SEPTEMBER 28

_____ _____ _____ _____ _____ _____ _____

SEPTEMBER 29–30

PERSONAL NOTES

SEPTEMBER 29, DAY OF THE WEEK　S　M　T　W　TH　F　S

	MOOD	VIGOR	SLEEP
Excellent			
	☐	☐	☐
	☐	☐	☐
	☐	☐	☐
Poor			

SEPTEMBER 30, DAY OF THE WEEK　S　M　T　W　TH　F　S

	MOOD	VIGOR	SLEEP
Excellent			
	☐	☐	☐
	☐	☐	☐
	☐	☐	☐
Poor			

NUTRITION LOG

	WHOLE GRAINS	FRUITS	VEGETABLES	PROTEIN	DAIRY	EXTRAS
GOALS (# SERVINGS)	3+	2+	3+	2–4	2–3	VARIABLE
SEPTEMBER 29	☐	☐	☐	☐	☐	☐
NOTES:						
SEPTEMBER 30	☐	☐	☐	☐	☐	☐
NOTES:						

CALCIUM + VITAMIN D ☐　VITAMIN E ☐　MULTIVITAMIN/MINERAL ☐

PLENTY OF FLUIDS ☐　OTHER SUPPLEMENTS _____

OVERALL COMMENTS

PHYSICAL ACTIVITY

planned, sport, leisure, errands, play
Goal: 30 to 60 minutes most days of the week

DAY	ACTIVITY	TIME

STRENGTH TRAINING

Goal: 2 to 3 times per week

EXERCISE 2 SETS/8 TO 10 REPS	DAY: POUNDS OR ✓	DAY: POUNDS OR ✓	DAY: POUNDS OR ✓

NUMBER OF STEPS

SEPTEMBER 29   SEPTEMBER 30

_____   _____

SEPTEMBER REVIEW

BRIGHT SPOTS:

_____

GREATEST CHALLENGES:

_____

_____

PATTERNS OBSERVED:

_____

IDENTIFY BARRIERS TO CHANGE AND HOW I AM GOING TO OVERCOME THEM:

    PERSONAL

_____

_____

    PROFESSIONAL

_____

_____

PERSONAL CARE ATTENTION (flossing teeth, skin care, cutting/coloring hair, etc.):

_____

_____

WELLNESS CHECK (Did I have any sick days?):

_____

_____

BODY WEIGHT: MONTHLY CYCLE DATES (if applicable):

_____

DOCTOR/DENTIST APPOINTMENTS:

_____

_____

MEDICATIONS TAKEN:

_____

_____

The Link Between Physical and Emotional Health

~❧~

Exercise "gives me both physical and spiritual strength," Sharon wrote to me. "I have overcome sadness by redoubling my efforts at fitness." In the research lab, we use terms like *self-efficacy* and *quality-of-life factors* to describe the emotional changes people experience as they become physically stronger. I like Sharon's way of explaining it better.

Countless other women have also written to me to tell me that increasing their physical strength led to increased emotional strength. The evidence isn't just anecdotal; it has been proven scientifically as well. In study after study on strength training completed at Tufts, we have found that exercise makes people feel empowered so that self-esteem and confidence soar. It is, in fact, one of our most robust findings. Even markers of depression in women have diminished significantly as they partake in an exercise program. In one research project at Tufts, colleagues of mine found that after just 10 weeks, depressed men and women who took part in a strength-training regimen experienced a two- to three-fold greater drop in depression than a similar group who did not lift weights.

I suspect much of the upswing in mood and outlook has to do with the fact that when you use your body in ways you never thought you could, the mind naturally follows suit. You realize that you *are* capable; that you do have control over your own life; that femininity is better expressed as the ability to do well by yourself rather than just accept life passively.

Dorothy, one of my favorite research volunteers, knows that as well as anyone. Now 75, she was 66 when she first joined one of my studies. Mother of 11 children and grandmother and great-grandmother to so many that I have lost count, she says the physical strength she has gained over the last decade (she now goes parasailing, surfing, and mountain biking) has given her the emotional strength she has needed to deal with whatever curves life has thrown her. Even better, it has made her joys all the more joyful.

October

OCTOBER 1–7

I have worked and volunteered in the fight against AIDS since the 1980s and have seen people at various stages of the disease. Some built their bodies from nothing into something after drug cocktails prolonged their lives. Others felt a sense of accomplishment just walking up the block. Still others didn't let their condition keep them from going back to school or seeking job retraining. And some stayed emotionally focused by making sure their children were taken care of. That's strength! That's also my inspiration. I am fortunate enough to be a relatively healthy woman. But when I do feel bad about myself, like most women do at one time or another, there is something that helps me stay strong: I do something for someone else. I can run up five flights of stairs to deliver a meal to a homebound person with AIDS, for instance. That's something I can do, and this boost of self-confidence shows me what I can accomplish.—MARY-SHANNON

PERSONAL NOTES

OCTOBER 1, DAY OF THE WEEK S M T W TH F S

MOOD	VIGOR	SLEEP
Excellent		
☐	☐	☐
☐	☐	☐
☐	☐	☐
Poor		

OCTOBER 2, DAY OF THE WEEK S M T W TH F S

MOOD	VIGOR	SLEEP
Excellent		
☐	☐	☐
☐	☐	☐
☐	☐	☐
Poor		

OCTOBER 3, DAY OF THE WEEK S M T W TH F S

MOOD	VIGOR	SLEEP
Excellent		
☐	☐	☐
☐	☐	☐
☐	☐	☐
Poor		

Sweet potato fries are delicious and more nutritious than regular French fries. To make them, coat a baking sheet with a thin layer of oil; peel sweet potatoes and cut into small wedges or strips; toss them on the baking sheet with a drop of oil, salt, and pepper; and bake at 450°F for about 25 minutes to a half hour. You can then drizzle them with a bit of balsamic vinegar if you'd like.

OCTOBER 4, DAY OF THE WEEK   S   M   T   W   TH   F   S

MOOD	VIGOR	SLEEP
Excellent		
☐	☐	☐
☐	☐	☐
☐	☐	☐
Poor		

OCTOBER 5, DAY OF THE WEEK   S   M   T   W   TH   F   S

MOOD	VIGOR	SLEEP
Excellent		
☐	☐	☐
☐	☐	☐
☐	☐	☐
Poor		

OCTOBER 6, DAY OF THE WEEK   S   M   T   W   TH   F   S

MOOD	VIGOR	SLEEP
Excellent		
☐	☐	☐
☐	☐	☐
☐	☐	☐
Poor		

OCTOBER 7, DAY OF THE WEEK   S   M   T   W   TH   F   S

MOOD	VIGOR	SLEEP
Excellent		
☐	☐	☐
☐	☐	☐
☐	☐	☐
Poor		

OCTOBER 1–7
NUTRITION LOG

	WHOLE GRAINS	FRUITS	VEGETABLES	PROTEIN	DAIRY	EXTRAS
GOALS (# SERVINGS)	3+	2+	3+	2–4	2–3	VARIABLE
OCTOBER 1	☐	☐	☐	☐	☐	☐
NOTES:						
OCTOBER 2	☐	☐	☐	☐	☐	☐
NOTES:						
OCTOBER 3	☐	☐	☐	☐	☐	☐
NOTES:						
OCTOBER 4	☐	☐	☐	☐	☐	☐
NOTES:						
OCTOBER 5	☐	☐	☐	☐	☐	☐
NOTES:						
OCTOBER 6	☐	☐	☐	☐	☐	☐
NOTES:						
OCTOBER 7	☐	☐	☐	☐	☐	☐
NOTES:						

CALCIUM + VITAMIN D ☐   VITAMIN E ☐   MULTIVITAMIN/MINERAL ☐

PLENTY OF FLUIDS ☐   OTHER SUPPLEMENTS _____

OVERALL COMMENTS

PHYSICAL ACTIVITY

planned, sport, leisure, errands, play
Goal: 30 to 60 minutes most days of the week

DAY	ACTIVITY	TIME

STRENGTH TRAINING

Goal: 2 to 3 times per week

EXERCISE 2 SETS/8 TO 10 REPS	DAY: POUNDS OR ✓	DAY: POUNDS OR ✓	DAY: POUNDS OR ✓

NUMBER OF STEPS

OCTOBER 1	OCTOBER 2	OCTOBER 3	OCTOBER 4	OCTOBER 5	OCTOBER 6	OCTOBER 7

OCTOBER 8–14

Strength comes from a variety of sources. As a motherless daughter, I was forced to find my inspiration from sources other than my mother. My role models for an adult woman were, of necessity, a composite of those women I encountered over the course of my life. Mostly my teachers, they gave me a sense of right and goodness that I have sought to maintain despite life's many obstacles. To nurture this strength and core of values, I have volunteered and continue to do so in service to others. The tutoring I do gives me a real sense of self-worth and of giving back to all those teachers who took an interest in me. I also find great inspiration by participating in various Race for the Cure events. Participating in the National Race for the Cure in Washington, D.C. this year gave me such a sense of awe that I was moved to tears.—SHARON

PERSONAL NOTES

OCTOBER 8, DAY OF THE WEEK   S   M   T   W   TH   F   S

MOOD	VIGOR	SLEEP
Excellent		
☐	☐	☐
☐	☐	☐
☐	☐	☐
Poor		

OCTOBER 9, DAY OF THE WEEK   S   M   T   W   TH   F   S

MOOD	VIGOR	SLEEP
Excellent		
☐	☐	☐
☐	☐	☐
☐	☐	☐
Poor		

OCTOBER 10, DAY OF THE WEEK   S   M   T   W   TH   F   S

MOOD	VIGOR	SLEEP
Excellent		
☐	☐	☐
☐	☐	☐
☐	☐	☐
Poor		

When you carry weights—or any other heavy objects—from one room or storage place to another, make sure to lift them properly. Squat down and lift only the amount of weight that you can lift easily, then stand up and move the equipment. Bending over at the hip and using your arms instead of your legs can cause strains and back injuries.

OCTOBER 11, DAY OF THE WEEK   S   M   T   W   TH   F   S

MOOD	VIGOR	SLEEP
Excellent		
☐	☐	☐
☐	☐	☐
☐	☐	☐
Poor		

OCTOBER 12, DAY OF THE WEEK   S   M   T   W   TH   F   S

MOOD	VIGOR	SLEEP
Excellent		
☐	☐	☐
☐	☐	☐
☐	☐	☐
Poor		

OCTOBER 13, DAY OF THE WEEK   S   M   T   W   TH   F   S

MOOD	VIGOR	SLEEP
Excellent		
☐	☐	☐
☐	☐	☐
☐	☐	☐
Poor		

OCTOBER 14, DAY OF THE WEEK   S   M   T   W   TH   F   S

MOOD	VIGOR	SLEEP
Excellent		
☐	☐	☐
☐	☐	☐
☐	☐	☐
Poor		

OCTOBER 8–14
NUTRITION LOG

GOALS (# SERVINGS)	WHOLE GRAINS 3+	FRUITS 2+	VEGETABLES 3+	PROTEIN 2–4	DAIRY 2–3	EXTRAS VARIABLE
OCTOBER 8 NOTES:	☐	☐	☐	☐	☐	☐
OCTOBER 9 NOTES:	☐	☐	☐	☐	☐	☐
OCTOBER 10 NOTES:	☐	☐	☐	☐	☐	☐
OCTOBER 11 NOTES:	☐	☐	☐	☐	☐	☐
OCTOBER 12 NOTES:	☐	☐	☐	☐	☐	☐
OCTOBER 13 NOTES:	☐	☐	☐	☐	☐	☐
OCTOBER 14 NOTES:	☐	☐	☐	☐	☐	☐

CALCIUM + VITAMIN D ☐   VITAMIN E ☐   MULTIVITAMIN/MINERAL ☐

PLENTY OF FLUIDS ☐   OTHER SUPPLEMENTS _____

OVERALL COMMENTS

PHYSICAL ACTIVITY

planned, sport, leisure, errands, play
Goal: 30 to 60 minutes most days of the week

DAY	ACTIVITY	TIME

STRENGTH TRAINING

Goal: 2 to 3 times per week

EXERCISE 2 SETS/8 TO 10 REPS	DAY: POUNDS OR ✓	DAY: POUNDS OR ✓	DAY: POUNDS OR ✓

NUMBER OF STEPS

OCTOBER 8	OCTOBER 9	OCTOBER 10	OCTOBER 11	OCTOBER 12	OCTOBER 13	OCTOBER 14

October 15–21

Doing something for someone else is just great. Some days it isn't a very big something. It could be picking up a neighbor's trash cover in the road or writing a note to someone I hardly know to wish them well. Just try looking for one small, helpful gesture each day. When you listen to your heart, it makes you a stronger woman.—DONNA

Personal Notes

OCTOBER 15, DAY OF THE WEEK S M T W TH F S

MOOD	VIGOR	SLEEP
Excellent		
☐	☐	☐
☐	☐	☐
☐	☐	☐
Poor		

OCTOBER 16, DAY OF THE WEEK S M T W TH F S

MOOD	VIGOR	SLEEP
Excellent		
☐	☐	☐
☐	☐	☐
☐	☐	☐
Poor		

OCTOBER 17, DAY OF THE WEEK S M T W TH F S

MOOD	VIGOR	SLEEP
Excellent		
☐	☐	☐
☐	☐	☐
☐	☐	☐
Poor		

Improve your body image—by exercising! Women who engage in regular physical activity have a better body image than other women—even if they weigh as many as 12 pounds more, according to a study in England. Maybe it's because the focus shifts from a few pounds that no one can see anyway to feeling stronger, more confident, and more in control. But also, regular exercisers look more toned than sedentary people, even with a few extra pounds on their frames.

OCTOBER 18, DAY OF THE WEEK   S   M   T   W   TH   F   S

MOOD	VIGOR	SLEEP
Excellent		
☐	☐	☐
☐	☐	☐
☐	☐	☐
Poor		

OCTOBER 19, DAY OF THE WEEK   S   M   T   W   TH   F   S

MOOD	VIGOR	SLEEP
Excellent		
☐	☐	☐
☐	☐	☐
☐	☐	☐
Poor		

OCTOBER 20, DAY OF THE WEEK   S   M   T   W   TH   F   S

MOOD	VIGOR	SLEEP
Excellent		
☐	☐	☐
☐	☐	☐
☐	☐	☐
Poor		

OCTOBER 21, DAY OF THE WEEK   S   M   T   W   TH   F   S

MOOD	VIGOR	SLEEP
Excellent		
☐	☐	☐
☐	☐	☐
☐	☐	☐
Poor		

OCTOBER 15–21
NUTRITION LOG

GOALS (# SERVINGS)	WHOLE GRAINS 3+	FRUITS 2+	VEGETABLES 3+	PROTEIN 2–4	DAIRY 2–3	EXTRAS VARIABLE
OCTOBER 15 NOTES:	☐	☐	☐	☐	☐	☐
OCTOBER 16 NOTES:	☐	☐	☐	☐	☐	☐
OCTOBER 17 NOTES:	☐	☐	☐	☐	☐	☐
OCTOBER 18 NOTES:	☐	☐	☐	☐	☐	☐
OCTOBER 19 NOTES:	☐	☐	☐	☐	☐	☐
OCTOBER 20 NOTES:	☐	☐	☐	☐	☐	☐
OCTOBER 21 NOTES:	☐	☐	☐	☐	☐	☐

CALCIUM + VITAMIN D ☐ VITAMIN E ☐ MULTIVITAMIN/MINERAL ☐

PLENTY OF FLUIDS ☐ OTHER SUPPLEMENTS _____

OVERALL COMMENTS

PHYSICAL ACTIVITY

planned, sport, leisure, errands, play
Goal: 30 to 60 minutes most days of the week

DAY	ACTIVITY	TIME

STRENGTH TRAINING

Goal: 2 to 3 times per week

EXERCISE 2 SETS/8 TO 10 REPS	DAY: POUNDS OR ✓	DAY: POUNDS OR ✓	DAY: POUNDS OR ✓

NUMBER OF STEPS

OCTOBER 15   OCTOBER 16   OCTOBER 17   OCTOBER 18   OCTOBER 19   OCTOBER 20   OCTOBER 21

_____   _____   _____   _____   _____   _____   _____

OCTOBER 22–28

I am active in my church to lighten my soul. I teach Sunday school to stay in touch with the pulse of our earth—our children.—PATTI

PERSONAL NOTES

OCTOBER 22, DAY OF THE WEEK   S   M   T   W   TH   F   S

MOOD	VIGOR	SLEEP
Excellent		
☐	☐	☐
☐	☐	☐
☐	☐	☐
Poor		

OCTOBER 23, DAY OF THE WEEK   S   M   T   W   TH   F   S

MOOD	VIGOR	SLEEP
Excellent		
☐	☐	☐
☐	☐	☐
☐	☐	☐
Poor		

OCTOBER 24, DAY OF THE WEEK   S   M   T   W   TH   F   S

MOOD	VIGOR	SLEEP
Excellent		
☐	☐	☐
☐	☐	☐
☐	☐	☐
Poor		

Need an excuse to do some more walking? Get a dog. It's a big responsibility, but research shows that people who have a dog tend to walk more than non-dog owners. (Their pets give them a great deal of pleasure and comfort, too.)

OCTOBER 25, DAY OF THE WEEK   S   M   T   W   TH   F   S

MOOD	VIGOR	SLEEP
Excellent		
Poor		

OCTOBER 26, DAY OF THE WEEK   S   M   T   W   TH   F   S

MOOD	VIGOR	SLEEP
Excellent		
Poor		

OCTOBER 27, DAY OF THE WEEK   S   M   T   W   TH   F   S

MOOD	VIGOR	SLEEP
Excellent		
Poor		

OCTOBER 28, DAY OF THE WEEK   S   M   T   W   TH   F   S

MOOD	VIGOR	SLEEP
Excellent		
Poor		

OCTOBER 22–28
NUTRITION LOG

GOALS (# SERVINGS)	WHOLE GRAINS	FRUITS	VEGETABLES	PROTEIN	DAIRY	EXTRAS
	3+	2+	3+	2–4	2–3	VARIABLE
OCTOBER 22	☐	☐	☐	☐	☐	☐
NOTES:						
OCTOBER 23	☐	☐	☐	☐	☐	☐
NOTES:						
OCTOBER 24	☐	☐	☐	☐	☐	☐
NOTES:						
OCTOBER 25	☐	☐	☐	☐	☐	☐
NOTES:						
OCTOBER 26	☐	☐	☐	☐	☐	☐
NOTES:						
OCTOBER 27	☐	☐	☐	☐	☐	☐
NOTES:						
OCTOBER 28	☐	☐	☐	☐	☐	☐
NOTES:						

CALCIUM + VITAMIN D ☐ VITAMIN E ☐ MULTIVITAMIN/MINERAL ☐

PLENTY OF FLUIDS ☐ OTHER SUPPLEMENTS _____

OVERALL COMMENTS

PHYSICAL ACTIVITY

planned, sport, leisure, errands, play
Goal: 30 to 60 minutes most days of the week

DAY	ACTIVITY	TIME

STRENGTH TRAINING

Goal: 2 to 3 times per week

EXERCISE 2 SETS/8 TO 10 REPS	DAY: POUNDS OR ✓	DAY: POUNDS OR ✓	DAY: POUNDS OR ✓

NUMBER OF STEPS

OCTOBER 22	OCTOBER 23	OCTOBER 24	OCTOBER 25	OCTOBER 26	OCTOBER 27	OCTOBER 28

OCTOBER 29–31

PERSONAL NOTES

OCTOBER 29, DAY OF THE WEEK   S   M   T   W   TH   F   S

MOOD	VIGOR	SLEEP
Excellent		
□	□	□
□	□	□
□	□	□
Poor		

OCTOBER 30, DAY OF THE WEEK   S   M   T   W   TH   F   S

MOOD	VIGOR	SLEEP
Excellent		
□	□	□
□	□	□
□	□	□
Poor		

OCTOBER 31, DAY OF THE WEEK   S   M   T   W   TH   F   S

MOOD	VIGOR	SLEEP
Excellent		
□	□	□
□	□	□
□	□	□
Poor		

OCTOBER 29–31
NUTRITION LOG

	WHOLE GRAINS	FRUITS	VEGETABLES	PROTEIN	DAIRY	EXTRAS
GOALS (# SERVINGS)	3+	2+	3+	2–4	2–3	VARIABLE
OCTOBER 29	☐	☐	☐	☐	☐	☐
NOTES:						
OCTOBER 30	☐	☐	☐	☐	☐	☐
NOTES:						
OCTOBER 31	☐	☐	☐	☐	☐	☐
NOTES:						

CALCIUM + VITAMIN D ☐ VITAMIN E ☐ MULTIVITAMIN/MINERAL ☐

PLENTY OF FLUIDS ☐ OTHER SUPPLEMENTS _____

OVERALL COMMENTS

PHYSICAL ACTIVITY

planned, sport, leisure, errands, play
Goal: 30 to 60 minutes most days of the week

DAY	ACTIVITY	TIME

STRENGTH TRAINING

Goal: 2 to 3 times per week

EXERCISE 2 SETS/8 TO 10 REPS	DAY: POUNDS OR ✓	DAY: POUNDS OR ✓	DAY: POUNDS OR ✓

NUMBER OF STEPS

OCTOBER 29   OCTOBER 30   OCTOBER 31

_____   _____   _____

OCTOBER REVIEW

BRIGHT SPOTS:

GREATEST CHALLENGES:

PATTERNS OBSERVED:

IDENTIFY BARRIERS TO CHANGE AND HOW I AM GOING TO OVERCOME THEM:

PERSONAL

PROFESSIONAL

PERSONAL CARE ATTENTION (flossing teeth, skin care, cutting/coloring hair, etc.):

WELLNESS CHECK (Did I have any sick days?):

BODY WEIGHT: MONTHLY CYCLE DATES (if applicable):

DOCTOR/DENTIST APPOINTMENTS:

MEDICATIONS TAKEN:

Becoming an Agent of Change

"I believe that in order to stay strong, it is important not only to take care of oneself but to give of oneself as well," Nancy wrote. That's why, in addition to being a volunteer mentor for teen parents, Nancy plans and organizes events for Leaders of Today & Tomorrow, a program that fosters leadership skills in young women.

Countless women have written to me expressing a similar sentiment. They feel that giving back, or acting as an agent of change for others, as I like to call it, offers them a spiritual strength that allows them to take care of themselves physically as well. Says Maryellen, a cardiac patient, "I participate in charity fundraising walks in my area, which gives me an opportunity to help others while taking care of myself. This type of service helps to balance me in the face of my daily challenges."

Indeed, it may even prolong life. A study from the University of Michigan found that, at least among older people, those who helped others reduced their risk of dying by more than half compared to their less giving peers.

Giving of yourself doesn't have to mean belonging to an organization. One woman, Cindy, told me of being "introduced by my best friend to road biking four years ago." It changed her life, allowing her to cope with the trials of going through difficult times with her son and deal with physical illness at a time that she felt spiritually bereft and just "exhausted from life."

"I had neglected myself for many years," Cindy wrote, but "I started to take my life back" with the help of the friend. The friend, of course, was Cindy's agent of change, and Cindy, in turn, was then able to pass on what she had been given. "I could give my found strength to others," she says. One way she does it: completing a 150-mile ride on her bike for multiple sclerosis!

November

November 1–7

I'm a human services coordinator, a wife, and a stepmother, and I have been overweight my whole life. My entire existence has been taking care of others, and I do it so well! I insist on a true familial atmosphere: full dinners prepared from scratch each night, quality family activities, participating and supporting each other in all aspects of life. It finally dawned on me—When do I get taken care of? Well, I went on strike. I laid it out for my family that I need them to share some of the work of our home life and that, until they did, I would do nothing. So a month went by with no meals, no cleaning, and no organizing. With all my free time, I invested in myself. I began eating so much better, I began exercising regularly, and I began socializing (I had lost touch with so many people). Now our whole life is happier and healthier, and we all take care of each other!—Rebecca

Personal Notes

NOVEMBER 1, DAY OF THE WEEK   S   M   T   W   TH   F   S

MOOD	VIGOR	SLEEP
Excellent		
☐	☐	☐
☐	☐	☐
☐	☐	☐
Poor		

NOVEMBER 2, DAY OF THE WEEK   S   M   T   W   TH   F   S

MOOD	VIGOR	SLEEP
Excellent		
☐	☐	☐
☐	☐	☐
☐	☐	☐
Poor		

NOVEMBER 3, DAY OF THE WEEK   S   M   T   W   TH   F   S

MOOD	VIGOR	SLEEP
Excellent		
☐	☐	☐
☐	☐	☐
☐	☐	☐
Poor		

You may have heard that *grilled, poached, roasted, and steamed* are good words to look for on a restaurant menu because they signify that a dish is low in fat. But that's not always the case. Sometimes chefs add butter or oil *after* cooking. Ask before ordering, and make your preference known.

NOVEMBER 4, DAY OF THE WEEK   S   M   T   W   TH   F   S

MOOD	VIGOR	SLEEP
Excellent		
☐	☐	☐
☐	☐	☐
☐	☐	☐
Poor		

NOVEMBER 5, DAY OF THE WEEK   S   M   T   W   TH   F   S

MOOD	VIGOR	SLEEP
Excellent		
☐	☐	☐
☐	☐	☐
☐	☐	☐
Poor		

NOVEMBER 6, DAY OF THE WEEK   S   M   T   W   TH   F   S

MOOD	VIGOR	SLEEP
Excellent		
☐	☐	☐
☐	☐	☐
☐	☐	☐
Poor		

NOVEMBER 7, DAY OF THE WEEK   S   M   T   W   TH   F   S

MOOD	VIGOR	SLEEP
Excellent		
☐	☐	☐
☐	☐	☐
☐	☐	☐
Poor		

NOVEMBER 1–7
NUTRITION LOG

	WHOLE GRAINS	FRUITS	VEGETABLES	PROTEIN	DAIRY	EXTRAS
GOALS (# SERVINGS)	3+	2+	3+	2–4	2–3	VARIABLE
NOVEMBER 1	☐	☐	☐	☐	☐	☐
NOTES:						
NOVEMBER 2	☐	☐	☐	☐	☐	☐
NOTES:						
NOVEMBER 3	☐	☐	☐	☐	☐	☐
NOTES:						
NOVEMBER 4	☐	☐	☐	☐	☐	☐
NOTES:						
NOVEMBER 5	☐	☐	☐	☐	☐	☐
NOTES:						
NOVEMBER 6	☐	☐	☐	☐	☐	☐
NOTES:						
NOVEMBER 7	☐	☐	☐	☐	☐	☐
NOTES:						

CALCIUM + VITAMIN D ☐ VITAMIN E ☐ MULTIVITAMIN/MINERAL ☐

PLENTY OF FLUIDS ☐ OTHER SUPPLEMENTS _____

OVERALL COMMENTS

PHYSICAL ACTIVITY

planned, sport, leisure, errands, play
Goal: 30 to 60 minutes most days of the week

DAY	ACTIVITY	TIME

STRENGTH TRAINING

Goal: 2 to 3 times per week

EXERCISE 2 SETS/8 TO 10 REPS	DAY: POUNDS OR ✓	DAY: POUNDS OR ✓	DAY: POUNDS OR ✓

NUMBER OF STEPS

NOVEMBER 1   NOVEMBER 2   NOVEMBER 3   NOVEMBER 4   NOVEMBER 5   NOVEMBER 6   NOVEMBER 7

November 8–14

Faced with an unlawful and unwarranted demotion at work, I filed a sex and age discrimination lawsuit against my employer. As a result, retaliation occurred in the workplace, and I had a nervous breakdown. The medicine prescribed left me like a zombie, along with sexual dysfunction. This was not for me. I then took a trial Tae Kwon Do lesson. I was desperate to rid myself of the anger that my boss had instilled in me. Through martial arts I was able to redirect my anger on the bags, breaking boards, and on my fellow martial arts students. Through martial arts, I also learned humility and perseverance. The intense workouts keep my body in shape and my endurance level that of a 22-year-old. The self-defense part, both physically and mentally, is the icing on the cake.—JUDITH

Personal Notes

NOVEMBER 8, DAY OF THE WEEK   S   M   T   W   TH   F   S

MOOD	VIGOR	SLEEP
Excellent		
☐	☐	☐
☐	☐	☐
☐	☐	☐
Poor		

NOVEMBER 9, DAY OF THE WEEK   S   M   T   W   TH   F   S

MOOD	VIGOR	SLEEP
Excellent		
☐	☐	☐
☐	☐	☐
☐	☐	☐
Poor		

NOVEMBER 10, DAY OF THE WEEK   S   M   T   W   TH   F   S

MOOD	VIGOR	SLEEP
Excellent		
☐	☐	☐
☐	☐	☐
☐	☐	☐
Poor		

Getting a massage may seem strictly like an indulgence, but it can also help reduce aches such as lower back pain. And it does feel good. A qualified masseuse (who can charge anywhere from about $45 to $120 an hour) will generally be certified by the National Certification Board for Therapeutic Massage and Bodywork or have graduated from a program approved by the Commission on Massage Therapy Accreditation.

NOVEMBER 11, DAY OF THE WEEK   S   M   T   W   TH   F   S

MOOD	VIGOR	SLEEP
Excellent		
☐	☐	☐
☐	☐	☐
☐	☐	☐
Poor		

NOVEMBER 12, DAY OF THE WEEK   S   M   T   W   TH   F   S

MOOD	VIGOR	SLEEP
Excellent		
☐	☐	☐
☐	☐	☐
☐	☐	☐
Poor		

NOVEMBER 13, DAY OF THE WEEK   S   M   T   W   TH   F   S

MOOD	VIGOR	SLEEP
Excellent		
☐	☐	☐
☐	☐	☐
☐	☐	☐
Poor		

NOVEMBER 14, DAY OF THE WEEK   S   M   T   W   TH   F   S

MOOD	VIGOR	SLEEP
Excellent		
☐	☐	☐
☐	☐	☐
☐	☐	☐
Poor		

November 8–14
Nutrition Log

GOALS (# SERVINGS)	WHOLE GRAINS 3+	FRUITS 2+	VEGETABLES 3+	PROTEIN 2–4	DAIRY 2–3	EXTRAS VARIABLE
NOVEMBER 8 NOTES:	☐	☐	☐	☐	☐	☐
NOVEMBER 9 NOTES:	☐	☐	☐	☐	☐	☐
NOVEMBER 10 NOTES:	☐	☐	☐	☐	☐	☐
NOVEMBER 11 NOTES:	☐	☐	☐	☐	☐	☐
NOVEMBER 12 NOTES:	☐	☐	☐	☐	☐	☐
NOVEMBER 13 NOTES:	☐	☐	☐	☐	☐	☐
NOVEMBER 14 NOTES:	☐	☐	☐	☐	☐	☐

CALCIUM + VITAMIN D ☐ **VITAMIN E** ☐ **MULTIVITAMIN/MINERAL** ☐

PLENTY OF FLUIDS ☐ **OTHER SUPPLEMENTS** _____

OVERALL COMMENTS

PHYSICAL ACTIVITY

planned, sport, leisure, errands, play
Goal: 30 to 60 minutes most days of the week

DAY	ACTIVITY	TIME

STRENGTH TRAINING

Goal: 2 to 3 times per week

EXERCISE 2 SETS/8 TO 10 REPS	DAY: POUNDS OR ✓	DAY: POUNDS OR ✓	DAY: POUNDS OR ✓

NUMBER OF STEPS

NOVEMBER 8   NOVEMBER 9   NOVEMBER 10   NOVEMBER 11   NOVEMBER 12   NOVEMBER 13   NOVEMBER 14

_____ _____ _____ _____ _____ _____ _____

November 15–21

As a physician, I have responsibilities to my patients and colleagues. As a woman, I have responsibilities to my family, friends, and community. I have come to realize that I have a responsibility to myself as well. The first step for me was the promise I made to myself when I started medical school. I had gradually lost 40 pounds throughout college and, knowing how hectic the lifestyle is during medical training, I vowed not to allow fitness to fall by the wayside and regain the weight. I've kept that promise one day at a time by packing healthy lunches, going for a run outside when the weather is nice, doing a Tae-Bo tape inside when it's not, and taking up Pilates when I need a change in routine. It's not about being selfish—it's about recognizing your own needs, attending to them, and building a stronger, healthier, and happier self that can then focus outward that much more effectively.—KRISTIN

Personal Notes

NOVEMBER 15, DAY OF THE WEEK S M T W TH F S

	MOOD	VIGOR	SLEEP
Excellent			
	☐	☐	☐
	☐	☐	☐
	☐	☐	☐
Poor			

NOVEMBER 16, DAY OF THE WEEK S M T W TH F S

	MOOD	VIGOR	SLEEP
Excellent			
	☐	☐	☐
	☐	☐	☐
	☐	☐	☐
Poor			

NOVEMBER 17, DAY OF THE WEEK S M T W TH F S

	MOOD	VIGOR	SLEEP
Excellent			
	☐	☐	☐
	☐	☐	☐
	☐	☐	☐
Poor			

If a stretch feels sharp or painful, you're doing it wrong. It should feel like a gentle pull. Breathe normally through every stretch. Holding your breath interrupts oxygen flow to your muscles.

NOVEMBER 18, DAY OF THE WEEK   S   M   T   W   TH   F   S

MOOD	VIGOR	SLEEP
Excellent		
Poor		

NOVEMBER 19, DAY OF THE WEEK   S   M   T   W   TH   F   S

MOOD	VIGOR	SLEEP
Excellent		
Poor		

NOVEMBER 20, DAY OF THE WEEK   S   M   T   W   TH   F   S

MOOD	VIGOR	SLEEP
Excellent		
Poor		

NOVEMBER 21, DAY OF THE WEEK   S   M   T   W   TH   F   S

MOOD	VIGOR	SLEEP
Excellent		
Poor		

November 15–21
NUTRITION LOG

	WHOLE GRAINS	FRUITS	VEGETABLES	PROTEIN	DAIRY	EXTRAS
GOALS (# SERVINGS)	3+	2+	3+	2–4	2–3	VARIABLE
NOVEMBER 15	☐	☐	☐	☐	☐	☐
NOTES:						
NOVEMBER 16	☐	☐	☐	☐	☐	☐
NOTES:						
NOVEMBER 17	☐	☐	☐	☐	☐	☐
NOTES:						
NOVEMBER 18	☐	☐	☐	☐	☐	☐
NOTES:						
NOVEMBER 19	☐	☐	☐	☐	☐	☐
NOTES:						
NOVEMBER 20	☐	☐	☐	☐	☐	☐
NOTES:						
NOVEMBER 21	☐	☐	☐	☐	☐	☐
NOTES:						

CALCIUM + VITAMIN D ☐   VITAMIN E ☐   MULTIVITAMIN/MINERAL ☐

PLENTY OF FLUIDS ☐   OTHER SUPPLEMENTS _____

OVERALL COMMENTS

PHYSICAL ACTIVITY

planned, sport, leisure, errands, play
Goal: 30 to 60 minutes most days of the week

DAY	ACTIVITY	TIME

STRENGTH TRAINING

Goal: 2 to 3 times per week

EXERCISE 2 SETS/8 TO 10 REPS	DAY: POUNDS OR ✓	DAY: POUNDS OR ✓	DAY: POUNDS OR ✓

NUMBER OF STEPS

NOVEMBER 15   NOVEMBER 16   NOVEMBER 17   NOVEMBER 18   NOVEMBER 19   NOVEMBER 20   NOVEMBER 21

_____   _____   _____   _____   _____   _____   _____

NOVEMBER 22–28

Others say that I'm too old to be running and that I should be eating whatever I want at my age. But as I get older I find that my health is the number-one thing in my life, for when I feel great, it affects my entire being and my attitude toward life and my family. Currently, I run three miles at least four to five mornings a week. I also exercise regularly with a power cord to build my arms, shoulders, legs, and back. Recently, I have lost 14 pounds (within two months) as a result of eating right (tons of veggies, fish, and chicken). I find I'm a much better person because of my daily regimen.—NANCY

PERSONAL NOTES

NOVEMBER 22, DAY OF THE WEEK S M T W TH F S

MOOD	VIGOR	SLEEP
Excellent		
☐	☐	☐
☐	☐	☐
☐	☐	☐
Poor		

NOVEMBER 23, DAY OF THE WEEK S M T W TH F S

MOOD	VIGOR	SLEEP
Excellent		
☐	☐	☐
☐	☐	☐
☐	☐	☐
Poor		

NOVEMBER 24, DAY OF THE WEEK S M T W TH F S

MOOD	VIGOR	SLEEP
Excellent		
☐	☐	☐
☐	☐	☐
☐	☐	☐
Poor		

Bagels are so big these days that even a plain one from a coffee shop chain without any butter or cream cheese has more calories than a jelly donut—about 350 versus 200, or the equivalent of eating five slices of white bread at a sitting. Better to grab a yogurt and slice of whole wheat bread from home that you can eat at the office.

NOVEMBER 25, DAY OF THE WEEK   S   M   T   W   TH   F   S

MOOD	VIGOR	SLEEP
Excellent		
☐	☐	☐
☐	☐	☐
☐	☐	☐
Poor		

NOVEMBER 26, DAY OF THE WEEK   S   M   T   W   TH   F   S

MOOD	VIGOR	SLEEP
Excellent		
☐	☐	☐
☐	☐	☐
☐	☐	☐
Poor		

NOVEMBER 27, DAY OF THE WEEK   S   M   T   W   TH   F   S

MOOD	VIGOR	SLEEP
Excellent		
☐	☐	☐
☐	☐	☐
☐	☐	☐
Poor		

NOVEMBER 28, DAY OF THE WEEK   S   M   T   W   TH   F   S

MOOD	VIGOR	SLEEP
Excellent		
☐	☐	☐
☐	☐	☐
☐	☐	☐
Poor		

NOVEMBER 22–28
NUTRITION LOG

	WHOLE GRAINS	FRUITS	VEGETABLES	PROTEIN	DAIRY	EXTRAS
GOALS (# SERVINGS)	3+	2+	3+	2–4	2–3	VARIABLE
NOVEMBER 22	☐	☐	☐	☐	☐	☐
NOTES:						
NOVEMBER 23	☐	☐	☐	☐	☐	☐
NOTES:						
NOVEMBER 24	☐	☐	☐	☐	☐	☐
NOTES:						
NOVEMBER 25	☐	☐	☐	☐	☐	☐
NOTES:						
NOVEMBER 26	☐	☐	☐	☐	☐	☐
NOTES:						
NOVEMBER 27	☐	☐	☐	☐	☐	☐
NOTES:						
NOVEMBER 28	☐	☐	☐	☐	☐	☐
NOTES:						

CALCIUM + VITAMIN D ☐   VITAMIN E ☐   MULTIVITAMIN/MINERAL ☐

PLENTY OF FLUIDS ☐   OTHER SUPPLEMENTS _____

OVERALL COMMENTS

PHYSICAL ACTIVITY

planned, sport, leisure, errands, play
Goal: 30 to 60 minutes most days of the week

DAY	ACTIVITY	TIME

STRENGTH TRAINING

Goal: 2 to 3 times per week

EXERCISE 2 SETS/8 TO 10 REPS	DAY: POUNDS OR ✓	DAY: POUNDS OR ✓	DAY: POUNDS OR ✓

NUMBER OF STEPS

NOVEMBER 22   NOVEMBER 23   NOVEMBER 24   NOVEMBER 25   NOVEMBER 26   NOVEMBER 27   NOVEMBER 28

November 29–30

Personal Notes

NOVEMBER 29, DAY OF THE WEEK S M T W TH F S

	MOOD	VIGOR	SLEEP
Excellent			
	☐	☐	☐
	☐	☐	☐
	☐	☐	☐
Poor			

NOVEMBER 30, DAY OF THE WEEK S M T W TH F S

	MOOD	VIGOR	SLEEP
Excellent			
	☐	☐	☐
	☐	☐	☐
	☐	☐	☐
Poor			

Nutrition Log

	WHOLE GRAINS	FRUITS	VEGETABLES	PROTEIN	DAIRY	EXTRAS
GOALS (# SERVINGS)	3+	2+	3+	2–4	2–3	VARIABLE
NOVEMBER 29	☐	☐	☐	☐	☐	☐
NOTES:						
NOVEMBER 30	☐	☐	☐	☐	☐	☐
NOTES:						

CALCIUM + VITAMIN D ☐ VITAMIN E ☐ MULTIVITAMIN/MINERAL ☐

PLENTY OF FLUIDS ☐ OTHER SUPPLEMENTS _____

OVERALL COMMENTS

PHYSICAL ACTIVITY

planned, sport, leisure, errands, play
Goal: 30 to 60 minutes most days of the week

DAY	ACTIVITY	TIME

STRENGTH TRAINING

Goal: 2 to 3 times per week

EXERCISE 2 SETS/8 TO 10 REPS	DAY: POUNDS OR ✓	DAY: POUNDS OR ✓	DAY: POUNDS OR ✓

NUMBER OF STEPS

NOVEMBER 29   NOVEMBER 30

_____   _____

NOVEMBER REVIEW

BRIGHT SPOTS:

_____

GREATEST CHALLENGES:

_____

_____

PATTERNS OBSERVED:

_____

IDENTIFY BARRIERS TO CHANGE AND HOW I AM GOING TO OVERCOME THEM:

    PERSONAL

_____

_____

    PROFESSIONAL

_____

_____

PERSONAL CARE ATTENTION (flossing teeth, skin care, cutting/coloring hair, etc.):

_____

_____

WELLNESS CHECK (Did I have any sick days?):

_____

_____

BODY WEIGHT: MONTHLY CYCLE DATES (if applicable):

_____

DOCTOR/DENTIST APPOINTMENTS:

_____

_____

MEDICATIONS TAKEN:

_____

_____

On Saying No (and Accepting Help)

❧

Growing up the only girl in a house of brothers, I was trained early to be accommodating. Sometimes I think we women are genetically programmed to bend over backward. In certain ways, it's a great trait, but eventually it can start to wear you down.

Since I turned 40, I have been working harder to limit how thin I spread myself out. It doesn't always feel comfortable to say "no," but I'm glad afterward. It allows me just a little extra time for the things I truly like to do.

Saying "no" isn't just about saying "no," however. It's also about saying "yes"—to help, to being more comfortable delegating tasks. You don't have to do everything yourself. During holidays, for instance, while the women in my family do all the cooking, I now get my husband and brothers well before mealtime to commit to doing the dishes afterward so that they don't disappear right after dinner. I'm not sure my husband is always totally thrilled with this new me, but he agrees it helps balance our relationship as well as our relationships with our children.

Saying no can also be used to overcome adversity. You make a decision that you're just not going to accept things the way they are, that you won't "wear" the limitations others try to impose on you. What happened to Jessica is a perfect example. Seventeen years ago, during a touch football game, she jumped for the ball and landed so hard, she says, that "my heel split in half, with the bone above lodged between the two halves. A doctor at the hospital said, 'This is a lifetime catastrophe.'" A physical therapist she worked with also thought she was going to live with severe limitations for life, but, comments Jessica, "It dawned on me that no one knew what was possible for me. I took on my own rehabilitation, and it worked!"

P.S. At 60, she's a competitive runner. How's that for "no"?

December

DECEMBER 1–7

*I was tired of being alone while my husband went on bike rides—so I decided to give it a try. Powered by my body, my mind, and my heart, I now ride a path to strength, health, and happiness. My bike takes me physically to incredibly beautiful places but also opens the door to intense recesses of strength and peace. In addition, my sport prompted an entire lifestyle change. I eat more nutritiously, exercise aerobically more often, and strength train—all to improve my biking abilities. As a result, I sleep better, look better, have increased energy, and enjoy a brighter outlook on life. The bigger bonus? I've met many wonderful people, and I have interests to share with my husband. A teacher once wrote on my homework, "Keep doing your best, but get out and play a little." More than 25 years later, I'm embracing that advice. The happiest people I know play often. I'm delighted to finally be among them.—*LISA

PERSONAL NOTES

DECEMBER 1, DAY OF THE WEEK S M T W TH F S

MOOD	VIGOR	SLEEP
Excellent		
□	□	□
□	□	□
□	□	□
Poor		

DECEMBER 2, DAY OF THE WEEK S M T W TH F S

MOOD	VIGOR	SLEEP
Excellent		
□	□	□
□	□	□
□	□	□
Poor		

DECEMBER 3, DAY OF THE WEEK S M T W TH F S

MOOD	VIGOR	SLEEP
Excellent		
□	□	□
□	□	□
□	□	□
Poor		

Don't grip the dumbbells too tightly when you are doing upper-body exercises. Yes, hold them with a full grip (including the thumbs), but don't clench. Your training will be more effective, not to mention more enjoyable.

DECEMBER 4, DAY OF THE WEEK S M T W TH F S

MOOD	VIGOR	SLEEP
Excellent		
Poor		

DECEMBER 5, DAY OF THE WEEK S M T W TH F S

MOOD	VIGOR	SLEEP
Excellent		
Poor		

DECEMBER 6, DAY OF THE WEEK S M T W TH F S

MOOD	VIGOR	SLEEP
Excellent		
Poor		

DECEMBER 7, DAY OF THE WEEK S M T W TH F S

MOOD	VIGOR	SLEEP
Excellent		
Poor		

DECEMBER 1–7
NUTRITION LOG

GOALS (# SERVINGS)	WHOLE GRAINS 3+	FRUITS 2+	VEGETABLES 3+	PROTEIN 2–4	DAIRY 2–3	EXTRAS VARIABLE
DECEMBER 1	☐	☐	☐	☐	☐	☐
NOTES:						
DECEMBER 2	☐	☐	☐	☐	☐	☐
NOTES:						
DECEMBER 3	☐	☐	☐	☐	☐	☐
NOTES:						
DECEMBER 4	☐	☐	☐	☐	☐	☐
NOTES:						
DECEMBER 5	☐	☐	☐	☐	☐	☐
NOTES:						
DECEMBER 6	☐	☐	☐	☐	☐	☐
NOTES:						
DECEMBER 7	☐	☐	☐	☐	☐	☐
NOTES:						

CALCIUM + VITAMIN D ☐   VITAMIN E ☐   MULTIVITAMIN/MINERAL ☐

PLENTY OF FLUIDS ☐   OTHER SUPPLEMENTS _____

OVERALL COMMENTS

PHYSICAL ACTIVITY

planned, sport, leisure, errands, play
Goal: 30 to 60 minutes most days of the week

DAY	ACTIVITY	TIME

STRENGTH TRAINING

Goal: 2 to 3 times per week

EXERCISE 2 SETS/8 TO 10 REPS	DAY: POUNDS OR ✓	DAY: POUNDS OR ✓	DAY: POUNDS OR ✓

NUMBER OF STEPS

DECEMBER 1   DECEMBER 2   DECEMBER 3   DECEMBER 4   DECEMBER 5   DECEMBER 6   DECEMBER 7

_____   _____   _____   _____   _____   _____   _____

December 8–14

Almost eight years ago, I was in a severe car accident and was told that I wouldn't ever be able to lift more than 20 pounds and would also have to give up doing certain things. But thanks to . . . determination and adding weight training to my routine, I am better than ever. For me, doing nothing but limiting my activities just didn't seem like an option.—Sonja

Personal Notes

DECEMBER 8, DAY OF THE WEEK   S   M   T   W   TH   F   S

MOOD	VIGOR	SLEEP
Excellent		
☐	☐	☐
☐	☐	☐
☐	☐	☐
Poor		

DECEMBER 9, DAY OF THE WEEK   S   M   T   W   TH   F   S

MOOD	VIGOR	SLEEP
Excellent		
☐	☐	☐
☐	☐	☐
☐	☐	☐
Poor		

DECEMBER 10, DAY OF THE WEEK   S   M   T   W   TH   F   S

MOOD	VIGOR	SLEEP
Excellent		
☐	☐	☐
☐	☐	☐
☐	☐	☐
Poor		

Eggplant, which tastes great grilled, is low on vitamins but also extremely low on calories—just 11 per half cup of 1-inch pieces. To keep calories low, brush it just very lightly with olive oil before grilling.

DECEMBER 11, DAY OF THE WEEK   S   M   T   W   TH   F   S

MOOD	VIGOR	SLEEP
Excellent		
☐	☐	☐
☐	☐	☐
☐	☐	☐
Poor		

DECEMBER 12, DAY OF THE WEEK   S   M   T   W   TH   F   S

MOOD	VIGOR	SLEEP
Excellent		
☐	☐	☐
☐	☐	☐
☐	☐	☐
Poor		

DECEMBER 13, DAY OF THE WEEK   S   M   T   W   TH   F   S

MOOD	VIGOR	SLEEP
Excellent		
☐	☐	☐
☐	☐	☐
☐	☐	☐
Poor		

DECEMBER 14, DAY OF THE WEEK   S   M   T   W   TH   F   S

MOOD	VIGOR	SLEEP
Excellent		
☐	☐	☐
☐	☐	☐
☐	☐	☐
Poor		

DECEMBER 8–14
NUTRITION LOG

GOALS (# SERVINGS)	WHOLE GRAINS 3+	FRUITS 2+	VEGETABLES 3+	PROTEIN 2–4	DAIRY 2–3	EXTRAS VARIABLE
DECEMBER 8	☐	☐	☐	☐	☐	☐
NOTES:						
DECEMBER 9	☐	☐	☐	☐	☐	☐
NOTES:						
DECEMBER 10	☐	☐	☐	☐	☐	☐
NOTES:						
DECEMBER 11	☐	☐	☐	☐	☐	☐
NOTES:						
DECEMBER 12	☐	☐	☐	☐	☐	☐
NOTES:						
DECEMBER 13	☐	☐	☐	☐	☐	☐
NOTES:						
DECEMBER 14	☐	☐	☐	☐	☐	☐
NOTES:						

CALCIUM + VITAMIN D ☐ VITAMIN E ☐ MULTIVITAMIN/MINERAL ☐

PLENTY OF FLUIDS ☐ OTHER SUPPLEMENTS _____

OVERALL COMMENTS

PHYSICAL ACTIVITY

planned, sport, leisure, errands, play
Goal: 30 to 60 minutes most days of the week

DAY	ACTIVITY	TIME

STRENGTH TRAINING

Goal: 2 to 3 times per week

EXERCISE 2 SETS/8 TO 10 REPS	DAY: POUNDS OR ✓	DAY: POUNDS OR ✓	DAY: POUNDS OR ✓

NUMBER OF STEPS

DECEMBER 8   DECEMBER 9   DECEMBER 10   DECEMBER 11   DECEMBER 12   DECEMBER 13   DECEMBER 14

_____   _____   _____   _____   _____   _____   _____

DECEMBER 15–21

My secret is to always remember, garbage in, garbage out. This is not just related to the obvious, like food choices, but also to the people, places, and things I surround myself with. I have a job I enjoy, where I feel productive and appreciated. I stay away from acquaintances who bring me down and instead focus on people who make me feel good and who I'm simply glad to know. I take the time to appreciate the important things in my life—my husband, puppy, family, and friends. I work out not because I have to but because it makes me feel empowered to know I'll live longer and healthier. I deliberately keep my life uncluttered by too many obligations. And I don't feel guilty about putting me first occasionally, or dabbling with garbage in. When put in perspective and practiced in moderation, a little indulgent behavior has its place. So if a hot fudge sundae is calling my name, or I take a long bubble bath instead of hitting the gym, so be it.—CHRISTINE

PERSONAL NOTES

DECEMBER 15, DAY OF THE WEEK   S   M   T   W   TH   F   S

MOOD	VIGOR	SLEEP
Excellent		
☐	☐	☐
☐	☐	☐
☐	☐	☐
Poor		

DECEMBER 16, DAY OF THE WEEK   S   M   T   W   TH   F   S

MOOD	VIGOR	SLEEP
Excellent		
☐	☐	☐
☐	☐	☐
☐	☐	☐
Poor		

DECEMBER 17, DAY OF THE WEEK   S   M   T   W   TH   F   S

MOOD	VIGOR	SLEEP
Excellent		
☐	☐	☐
☐	☐	☐
☐	☐	☐
Poor		

Stick to a plan of limiting yourself to no more than one hour of television a day. If you turn off the set, you're bound to use your body more to do errands—or at least exercise your brain by reading a little. You'll cut down on TV-time snacking, too.

DECEMBER 18, DAY OF THE WEEK   S   M   T   W   TH   F   S

MOOD	VIGOR	SLEEP
Excellent		
☐	☐	☐
☐	☐	☐
☐	☐	☐
Poor		

DECEMBER 19, DAY OF THE WEEK   S   M   T   W   TH   F   S

MOOD	VIGOR	SLEEP
Excellent		
☐	☐	☐
☐	☐	☐
☐	☐	☐
Poor		

DECEMBER 20, DAY OF THE WEEK   S   M   T   W   TH   F   S

MOOD	VIGOR	SLEEP
Excellent		
☐	☐	☐
☐	☐	☐
☐	☐	☐
Poor		

DECEMBER 21, DAY OF THE WEEK   S   M   T   W   TH   F   S

MOOD	VIGOR	SLEEP
Excellent		
☐	☐	☐
☐	☐	☐
☐	☐	☐
Poor		

DECEMBER 15–21
NUTRITION LOG

GOALS (# SERVINGS)	WHOLE GRAINS 3+	FRUITS 2+	VEGETABLES 3+	PROTEIN 2–4	DAIRY 2–3	EXTRAS VARIABLE
DECEMBER 15 NOTES:	☐	☐	☐	☐	☐	☐
DECEMBER 16 NOTES:	☐	☐	☐	☐	☐	☐
DECEMBER 17 NOTES:	☐	☐	☐	☐	☐	☐
DECEMBER 18 NOTES:	☐	☐	☐	☐	☐	☐
DECEMBER 19 NOTES:	☐	☐	☐	☐	☐	☐
DECEMBER 20 NOTES:	☐	☐	☐	☐	☐	☐
DECEMBER 21 NOTES:	☐	☐	☐	☐	☐	☐

CALCIUM + VITAMIN D ☐   VITAMIN E ☐   MULTIVITAMIN/MINERAL ☐

PLENTY OF FLUIDS ☐   OTHER SUPPLEMENTS _____

OVERALL COMMENTS

PHYSICAL ACTIVITY

planned, sport, leisure, errands, play
Goal: 30 to 60 minutes most days of the week

DAY	ACTIVITY	TIME

STRENGTH TRAINING

Goal: 2 to 3 times per week

EXERCISE 2 SETS/8 TO 10 REPS	DAY: POUNDS OR ✓	DAY: POUNDS OR ✓	DAY: POUNDS OR ✓

NUMBER OF STEPS

DECEMBER 15   DECEMBER 16   DECEMBER 17   DECEMBER 18   DECEMBER 19   DECEMBER 20   DECEMBER 21

_____   _____   _____   _____   _____   _____   _____

DECEMBER 22–28

When you are young, you exercise to lose weight, to look good, and because everyone else does it. When you get older, you exercise to live, to move without pain, and to stay free and independent. You have, by this time, defined your territory, and you know that you must defend it and hope to expand it. And that only happens if you are strong. So you stay focused and keep trying. Some things work. Some are a waste of time. Some you stay with forever. Whatever—just keep moving, evaluating. Things always change.—LINDA

PERSONAL NOTES

DECEMBER 22, DAY OF THE WEEK   S   M   T   W   TH   F   S

MOOD	VIGOR	SLEEP
Excellent		
☐	☐	☐
☐	☐	☐
☐	☐	☐
Poor		

DECEMBER 23, DAY OF THE WEEK   S   M   T   W   TH   F   S

MOOD	VIGOR	SLEEP
Excellent		
☐	☐	☐
☐	☐	☐
☐	☐	☐
Poor		

DECEMBER 24, DAY OF THE WEEK   S   M   T   W   TH   F   S

MOOD	VIGOR	SLEEP
Excellent		
☐	☐	☐
☐	☐	☐
☐	☐	☐
Poor		

Allow yourself to believe in yourself. It has been shown numerous times that people who *believe* they can get fit and eat well are more successful at achieving these behavioral changes than people who don't believe in themselves.

DECEMBER 25, DAY OF THE WEEK   S   M   T   W   TH   F   S

MOOD	VIGOR	SLEEP
Excellent		
☐	☐	☐
☐	☐	☐
☐	☐	☐
Poor		

DECEMBER 26, DAY OF THE WEEK   S   M   T   W   TH   F   S

MOOD	VIGOR	SLEEP
Excellent		
☐	☐	☐
☐	☐	☐
☐	☐	☐
Poor		

DECEMBER 27, DAY OF THE WEEK   S   M   T   W   TH   F   S

MOOD	VIGOR	SLEEP
Excellent		
☐	☐	☐
☐	☐	☐
☐	☐	☐
Poor		

DECEMBER 28, DAY OF THE WEEK   S   M   T   W   TH   F   S

MOOD	VIGOR	SLEEP
Excellent		
☐	☐	☐
☐	☐	☐
☐	☐	☐
Poor		

DECEMBER 22–28
NUTRITION LOG

GOALS (# SERVINGS)	WHOLE GRAINS 3+	FRUITS 2+	VEGETABLES 3+	PROTEIN 2–4	DAIRY 2–3	EXTRAS VARIABLE
DECEMBER 22	☐	☐	☐	☐	☐	☐
NOTES:						
DECEMBER 23	☐	☐	☐	☐	☐	☐
NOTES:						
DECEMBER 24	☐	☐	☐	☐	☐	☐
NOTES:						
DECEMBER 25	☐	☐	☐	☐	☐	☐
NOTES:						
DECEMBER 26	☐	☐	☐	☐	☐	☐
NOTES:						
DECEMBER 27	☐	☐	☐	☐	☐	☐
NOTES:						
DECEMBER 28	☐	☐	☐	☐	☐	☐
NOTES:						

CALCIUM + VITAMIN D ☐ VITAMIN E ☐ MULTIVITAMIN/MINERAL ☐

PLENTY OF FLUIDS ☐ OTHER SUPPLEMENTS _____

OVERALL COMMENTS

PHYSICAL ACTIVITY

planned, sport, leisure, errands, play
Goal: 30 to 60 minutes most days of the week

DAY	ACTIVITY	TIME

STRENGTH TRAINING

Goal: 2 to 3 times per week

EXERCISE 2 SETS/8 TO 10 REPS	DAY: POUNDS OR ✓	DAY: POUNDS OR ✓	DAY: POUNDS OR ✓

NUMBER OF STEPS

DECEMBER 22   DECEMBER 23   DECEMBER 24   DECEMBER 25   DECEMBER 26   DECEMBER 27   DECEMBER 28

_____   _____   _____   _____   _____   _____   _____

DECEMBER 29–31

PERSONAL NOTES

DECEMBER 29, DAY OF THE WEEK   S   M   T   W   TH   F   S

MOOD	VIGOR	SLEEP
	Excellent	
☐	☐	☐
☐	☐	☐
☐	☐	☐
	Poor	

DECEMBER 30, DAY OF THE WEEK   S   M   T   W   TH   F   S

MOOD	VIGOR	SLEEP
	Excellent	
☐	☐	☐
☐	☐	☐
☐	☐	☐
	Poor	

DECEMBER 31, DAY OF THE WEEK   S   M   T   W   TH   F   S

MOOD	VIGOR	SLEEP
	Excellent	
☐	☐	☐
☐	☐	☐
☐	☐	☐
	Poor	

DECEMBER 29–31
NUTRITION LOG

GOALS (# SERVINGS)	WHOLE GRAINS 3+	FRUITS 2+	VEGETABLES 3+	PROTEIN 2–4	DAIRY 2–3	EXTRAS VARIABLE
DECEMBER 29	☐	☐	☐	☐	☐	☐
NOTES:						
DECEMBER 30	☐	☐	☐	☐	☐	☐
NOTES:						
DECEMBER 31	☐	☐	☐	☐	☐	☐
NOTES:						

CALCIUM + VITAMIN D ☐   VITAMIN E ☐   MULTIVITAMIN/MINERAL ☐

PLENTY OF FLUIDS ☐   OTHER SUPPLEMENTS _____

OVERALL COMMENTS

PHYSICAL ACTIVITY

planned, sport, leisure, errands, play
Goal: 30 to 60 minutes most days of the week

DAY	ACTIVITY	TIME

STRENGTH TRAINING

Goal: 2 to 3 times per week

EXERCISE 2 SETS/8 TO 10 REPS	DAY: POUNDS OR ✓	DAY: POUNDS OR ✓	DAY: POUNDS OR ✓

NUMBER OF STEPS

DECEMBER 29   DECEMBER 30   DECEMBER 31

_____   _____   _____

DECEMBER REVIEW

BRIGHT SPOTS:
_____

GREATEST CHALLENGES:
_____
_____
_____

PATTERNS OBSERVED:
_____
_____

IDENTIFY BARRIERS TO CHANGE AND HOW I AM GOING TO OVERCOME THEM:

    PERSONAL
_____
_____

    PROFESSIONAL
_____
_____

PERSONAL CARE ATTENTION (flossing teeth, skin care, cutting/coloring hair, etc.):
_____
_____

WELLNESS CHECK (Did I have any sick days?):
_____
_____

BODY WEIGHT: MONTHLY CYCLE DATES (if applicable):
_____

DOCTOR/DENTIST APPOINTMENTS:
_____
_____

MEDICATIONS TAKEN:
_____
_____
_____

Seasons

❦

"In 1995," writes Sally, "I moved from being a ski instructor to marketing management. The change from constant activity to desk-driving meant a rapid gain of more than 60 pounds. I also missed being outside—winters on the slopes and summers on my bike or hiking. Finally, about a year ago, I reached a point where I knew something had to give. I tried to change my diet and exercise, though it was difficult to avoid the greasy food served in the restaurant at work, and exercising indoors felt like a chore. Then I bought a pair of snowshoes. What a difference! Instead of dreading exercise, I couldn't wait to get outside in the fresh air. Being active motivated me to eat better. Then, in spring, I sprang for a kayak."

I know just where Sally is coming from. The seasons make a big difference to me as well. And I try to make the most of them. In the spring I stop by our local farm stand every day to buy freshly picked asparagus; in summer I pick up corn on the cob, and we grill something almost every night. In the late fall I am a fan of beets and winter squash.

I also adapt my exercise habits to the seasons, as Sally does. Summertime means running, hiking, and swimming. In the fall I do more biking. And during winter and early spring I cross-country ski and ice skate, and I rock climb indoors!

I also like to sleep a little longer in the winter. I don't know whether it's the feel of a warm, comfortable bed when it's cold outside or a true seasonal swing in my body's needs. But I do try to go with the seasonal flow. I love the variety in lifestyle that the seasons encourage, and I think it helps me stay active and motivated. I hope you take advantage of the seasons to live a richer life, too.

Keeping Yourself Well: Medical Screenings

Everyone should go for a physical once a year as a matter of course. It's important to check in with your doctor even if you feel perfectly fine so that she or he can run some routine screening tests to check your health from the inside out.

Which medical screenings to get at which stage of life can be very confusing—because the age at which each one is appropriate can be a moving target. Are you supposed to get a mammogram every year starting at 40? Every other year? What about Pap smears to check for cervical cancer?

Part of determining which tests and when to have them depends on the state of your health to begin with. For instance, it is generally recommended that a woman get a pelvic exam and a Pap smear every two to three years—but only if she has had three exams three years in a row that have come up negative. Bone density measurements are not covered by health insurance in most cases until a woman is 65, but many health professionals (including me) believe all women should get a baseline scan around the time of menopause so that, if need be, aggressive measures can be taken against osteoporosis when there's still time to do something about it.

Following is a list of medical screenings every woman should get at some point. Where I can, I give the generally accepted guidelines for when—or how often—the screening should occur. Take this list with you to your annual physical because the guidelines are always changing. More to the point, everyone's different. You should go over the items with your doctor to make sure you're getting the right tests at the right time of *your* life.

SCREENING TESTS

Blood pressure Every physician visit, or at least every one to two years.

Blood cholesterol Every five years, at least through age 65.

Physician breast exam Annually for women over 40.

Mammogram The American Cancer Society recommends annual mammograms for all women beginning at age 40. The National Cancer Institute advises women over 40 to get one every one to two years.

Pelvic exam and Pap smear Every two to three years after three years in a row of negative results. Less often after age 65 *unless* regular screening has not been done in the past.

Digital rectal exam (to check for colon cancer) Once a year after age 40.

Fecal Occult [Hidden] Blood Test (to check for colon cancer) Once a year after age 50.

Colonoscopy Every 10 years starting at age 50, unless otherwise advised by your doctor.

Electrocardiogram (records the heart's rhythms) The American Heart Association recommends periodic electrocardiograms after age 40.

Sensitive TSH (Thyroid Stimulating Hormone) Test (checks for thyroid dysfunction) Every 5 years, starting at age 35.

Bone Density Scan The official recommendations are for every woman to have a bone density test every 2 to 5 years starting at age 65. If possible, I recommend that a woman get a bone density scan at the time of menopause so that she can learn her baseline bone density and take extra precautions if needed.

Dental checkup Twice a year.

Dermatologist visit to check for skin cancer Discuss advisability and frequency with your primary care physician.

Eye exam Annually. Includes measurement of intraocular pressure to check for glaucoma.

IMMUNIZATIONS

Flu vaccine Advised annually for people over 65.

Pneumonia vaccine Anyone given the vaccine before age 65 should be re-immunized upon turning 65 if more than six years have passed since the initial shot. Anyone over 65 who has never received it should get one.

Tetanus-diphtheria vaccine Every 10 years throughout life.

A YEAR IN REVIEW

ONCE A YEAR IT'S A GOOD IDEA to sit down for an hour or two and assess the progress you have made as well as set new goals, or reset old ones. You will see that many of the things I ask you to consider echo what you've been asked to assess on a monthly basis. But looking things over from month to month, as you have been doing, should make it much easier to consider how things have gone over the year as a whole.

Filling out these pages will let you see very quickly where you've accomplished what you set out to do, where you might want to retrench, and what obstacles you need to get around as you move forward.

For those goals you've reached, pat yourself on the back. For those you haven't achieved yet, never, never beat yourself up. Life is a process, not an endpoint. Take all your experience as learning tools, and proceed with confidence.

Yearly Check List

DATE _____

NUTRITION

Did I meet the basic nutrition goals? ☐ Yes ☐ No

Goals that I achieved most days of the week:

Whole grains (3+)   Fruits (2+)   Vegetables (3+)   Protein (2–4)   Dairy (2–3)

Was my attitude toward food and nutrition flexible? ☐ Yes ☐ No

What supplements did I take on a regular basis? _____

_____

What do I need to work on most to meet my nutrition goals for overall health?

_____

_____

_____

_____

EXERCISE

Did I meet the basic exercise goals? ☐ Yes ☐ No

Physical activity:

Goals that I achieved:

5 to 7 sessions per week   30 or more minutes per day

Average number of steps per day: _____

Types of physical activity: _____

_____

Strength training:

Goals that I achieved:

2 to 3 sessions per week   6 to 9 exercises per session

Did I increase the amount of weight that I lifted over the year? ☐ Yes ☐ No

Did I stretch after each workout? ☐ Yes ☐ No

General:

Did I experience any injuries related to exercise? ☐ Yes ☐ No

If yes, what type of injury, and how was it treated?_____

_____

What do I need to work on most to meet my exercise goals for overall health?

_____

_____

_____

_____

BODY WEIGHT AND HEIGHT

My height and weight (in the morning)

Height: _____   Weight: _____

Over the year, what was my:

Lowest weight? _____ Highest weight? _____

My goal weight: _____

Do I want to lose weight? If so, how much? _____

Am I committed to losing weight slowly and in a healthy way? ☐ Yes ☐ No

What safe and reasonable weight-loss steps am I prepared to take?

_____

_____

_____

MEDICAL CHECKUP

Medical conditions (new or chronic; issues around monthly cycle; etc.):

_____

_____

_____

Medications taken:

_____

_____

_____

Diagnostic tests taken:

_____

_____

_____

Significant findings

_____

_____

Immunizations received

_____

_____

MOOD, VIGOR AND SLEEP

Overall, how was my:

Mood?   _____

Vigor?   _____

Sleep?   _____

LIFESTYLE

Are there any lifestyle concerns that I want to address next year, such as smoking, drinking, stress, relationships? ☐ Yes ☐ No

If yes, what are they and how do I plan to work on them?

_____

_____

_____

Greatest accomplishments for the year:

_____

_____

_____

Greatest challenges:

_____

_____

_____

What months were best?   _____

What months were most difficult? _____

Patterns observed: _____

_____

What strategies from months that went well could I transfer to the more difficult months?

_____

_____

Identify next year's major goals:

Nutrition _____

How am I going to accomplish them? _____

Physical activity _____

How am I going to accomplish them?

_____

_____

_____

Personal _____

How am I going to accomplish them?

_____

_____

_____

Professional _____

How am I going to accomplish them?

_____

_____

_____

Resources

THE FOLLOWING SOURCES WILL HELP YOU MEET nutrition and exercise goals—*soundly*.

Strong Women Books, Video and Website

Strong Women Stay Young (Bantam Books), by Miriam E. Nelson, Ph.D., with Sarah Wernick, Ph.D. Provides a basic strength training program for women of all ages to help replace fat with muscle, reverse bone loss, and improve energy and balance. Called "an essential tool for women of all ages" by C. Everett Koop, M.D., the former Surgeon General.

Strong Women Stay Slim (Bantam Books), by Miriam E. Nelson, Ph.D., with Sarah Wernick, Ph.D. An exercise and eating plan for shedding fat, firming the body, and boosting metabolism—without deprivation. The editor-in-chief of *Shape* magazine, Barbara Harris, refers to it as "thoroughly based in science yet written to help women get started immediately to make their lives better today."

Strong Women, Strong Bones (G.P. Putnam's Sons), by Miriam E. Nelson, Ph.D., with Sarah Wernick, Ph.D. Everything you need to know to prevent as well as treat osteoporosis, from exercise to diet (it's not just calcium) to medications beyond hormone replacement therapy. "Comprehensive information . . . makes Dr. Nelson's book an excellent resource to help women . . . achieve optimal bone health, regardless of their age," says Sandra C. Raymond, the chief executive director of the National Osteoporosis Foundation.

Strong Women Eat Well (G.P. Putnam's Sons), by Miriam E. Nelson, Ph.D., with Judy Knipe. Easy-to-follow strategies for incorporating healthful foods into a busy lifestyle with advice on dietary supplements and 50 delicious recipes. Irwin H. Rosenberg, M.D., Dean of the Friedman School of Nutrition Science and Policy at Tufts University, says it "is scientifically sound, full of nutritional strategies that are easy to follow, and clearly written. This is essential reading for every woman."

Strong Women and Men Beat Arthritis (G.P. Putnam's Sons), by Miriam E. Nelson, Ph.D., Kristin R. Baker, Ph.D., and Ronenn Roubenoff, M.D., M.H.S., with Lawrence Lindner, M.A. Cutting-edge strategies for the relief of both osteoarthritis and rheumatoid arthritis. Allows people with arthritis to reduce pain and disability as well as improve mood and boost self-confidence. Nancy L. Snyderman, M.D., medical correspondent for ABC News, says the book "should be in the hands of people struggling with arthritis—and also in the hands of their doctors."

The Strong Women Stay Young Video A real-time exercise video focusing on strength training based on my first book is available from www.healthletter.tufts.edu, or call (800) 203-5585. You can also order this video through www.aswechange.com.

Strongwomen.com I developed this website to provide women (and men) information regarding nutrition and exercise. In addition, you can sign up for a free, monthly electronic newsletter that provides updates on research, my speaking engagements, and other tips and recipes that you can easily use.

Tufts University Resources

Tufts University Health & Nutrition Letter This monthly, 8-page newsletter has been called "the best available source of news and views on nutrition" by *U.S. News & World Report*. It has also received accolades from *The New York Times, Cooking Light* magazine, the *Columbia Journalism Review*, and many other publications. You can also order my books and video from the *Letter*. To order, call (800) 274-7581 or surf to www.healthletter.tufts.edu.

Navigator.tufts.edu A Tufts website that evaluates the accuracy and perspective of the nutrition information posted on hundreds of sites across the Internet, Navigator "hacks through this jungle of hype to help users quickly find trustworthy nutrition information," according to *Brill's Content*. It has also been lauded by the *Journal of the American Medical Association* as well as newspapers across the country.

Where to Buy a Pedometer

Most sporting goods stores carry a variety of pedometers that count steps and distance walked throughout the day. You can purchase a pedometer online at www.thepedometercompany.com (telephone: 1-888-748-5377 or 1-816-353-1721). A good brand is Digiwalker. Most pedometers cost between $20 and $30. There is no need to buy a fancy one that sings and counts calories. The most important thing is that it accurately counts your steps.

Organizations

American Council on Exercise
4851 Paramount Drive
San Diego, CA 92123
(800) 825-3636
www.acefitness.org
A fitness organization where you can locate a certified exercise professional in your area.

American College of Sports Medicine
P.O. Box 1440
Indianapolis, IN 46206
www.acsm.org
An organization that facilitates research in the field of exercise science as well as certifies fitness professionals.

American Dietetics Association (ADA)
216 West Jackson Boulevard
Chicago, IL 60606-6995
(800) 366-1655
www.eatright.org
Features comprehensive nutrition information for the public, including a database of dietitians in your area.

Arthritis Foundation
P.O. Box 7669
Atlanta, GA 30357-0669
(800) 283-7800

www.arthritis.org
Comprehensive information for preventing and treating arthritis.

Centers for Disease Control and Prevention
National Center for Chronic Disease Prevention and Health Promotion (NCCDPHP)
4770 Buford Hwy, NE
Atlanta, GA 30341-3717
www.cdc.gov/nccdphp
Division of Nutrition and Physical Activity (DNPA)
www.cdc.gov/nccdphp/dnpa
Offers information about nutrition, physical activity, and numerous other health-related topics.

Fifty-Plus Fitness Association
P.O. Box 20230
Stanford, CA 94309
(650) 323-6160
www.50plus.org
An organization whose sole mission is the promotion of physical activity for older adults.

National Strength and Conditioning Association
1640 L St. Suite G
Lincoln, NE 68508
(888) 746-2378
www.nsca-lift.org
An organization where you can locate a certified fitness professional in your geographical area.

National Osteoporosis Foundation
1150 17th St. N.W., Suite 500
Washington, DC 20036
(202) 223-2226
www.nof.org
Comprehensive information for preventing and treating osteoporosis.

Shape-Up America!
6707 Democracy Boulevard, Suite 306
Bethesda, MD 20817
(301) 493-5368
www.shapeup.org
Information about weight control and other health-related topics.

Books

Biomarkers: The 10 Determinants of Aging You Can Control, by William Evans, Ph.D.
and Irwin Rosenberg, M.D., with Jacqueline Thompson (Simon & Schulster, 1991)
Strength Training Past 50, by Wayne Wescott, Ph.D. (Human Kinetics, 1997)

Equipment

All Pro Exercise Products, Inc.
P.O. Box 8268
Longboat Key, FL 34228
(800) 735-9287
www.allproweights.com

Australian Barbell Company
54 Bond Street West
Mordialloc 3195
Melbourne, Victoria
Australia
Phone: (03) 9580 5945
Fax: (03) 9580 7123
www.australianbarbellco.com

Keiser Sports Health Equipment
2470 South Cherry Avenue
Fresno, CA 93706
(800) 888-7009
(559) 256-8000
www.keiser.com

❧
About the Author

MIRIAM E. NELSON, PH.D., IS DIRECTOR OF the John Hancock Center for Physical Activity and Nutrition and Associate Professor of Nutrition at the Friedman School of Nutrition Science and Policy at Tufts University. She is also a fellow of the American College of Sports Medicine, an honor reserved for those who have demonstrated superior leadership and research in the field of exercise.

For the last 15 years, Dr. Nelson has been principal investigator of studies on exercise and nutrition for older adults, work supported by grants from the government and private foundations. During this time she was named a Brookdale National Fellow, a prestigious award given annually to only five or six young scholars deemed to be future leaders in the field of aging. She was also awarded a Bunting Fellowship at the Mary Ingraham Bunting Institute at Radcliffe College. In 1998, Dr. Nelson received the Lifetime Achievement Award from the Massachusetts Governor's Committee on Physical Fitness and Sports.

Dr. Nelson is the author of five international best-sellers: *Strong Women Stay Young; Strong Women Stay Slim; Strong Women, Strong Bones; Strong Women Eat Well*; and *Strong Women and Men Beat Arthritis*. These titles, published in 13 languages, have collectively sold more than a million copies worldwide. *Strong Women, Strong Bones* received the esteemed Books for a Better Life Award for best wellness book of 2000 from the Multiple Sclerosis Society.

In August 2001, Dr. Nelson appeared in her own PBS special entitled *Strong Women Live Well*, which focused on the benefits of exercise and nutrition for women's health. She has been featured on many television and radio shows, including *The Oprah Winfrey Show, The Today Show, Good Morning America,* and *Fresh Air,* as well as on CNN and the Discovery Channel. She is also a motivational speaker who lectures about women's health around the world.

She lives in Concord, Massachusetts, with her husband and three children.

To contact Dr. Nelson, please send letters to:
Miriam E. Nelson, Ph.D.
Friedman School of Nutrition Science and Policy at Tufts University
150 Harrison Avenue
Boston, MA 02111
www.strongwomen.com

Dr. Nelson regrets that due to the volume of mail she receives, she cannot respond personally to every letter.

NOTES